The Essential Guide to the New FRCR Part 1

Tony Jeswani
Registrar in Radiology
Royal Free Hospital, London

and

John Morlese
Specialist Registrar in Radiology
Royal Free Hospital, London

Foreword by

Andrew Platts
Consultant Vascular and Neuroradiologist
Royal Free Hospital, London

Radcliffe Publishing

Oxford ● Seattle

Radcliffe Publishing Ltd
18 Marcham Road
Abingdon
Oxon OX14 1AA
United Kingdom

www.radcliffe-oxford.com
Electronic catalogue and worldwide online ordering facility.

British Library Cataloguing in Publication Data

A catalogue record for this book is available from the British Library.

ISBN 1 85775 616 9

Typeset by Advance Typesetting Ltd, Oxford
Printed and bound by TJ International Ltd, Padstow, Cornwall

Contents

Foreword

The new FRCR Part 1 has brought with it a new curriculum and is examined using a multiple choice format.

Multiple choice examination has been shown to be a fair way of assessing the knowledge and problem-solving ability of candidates. It is also extremely useful as a teaching tool. It is very difficult when setting multiple choice questions to produce plausible, yet demonstrably incorrect, negative answers. Those of you who have not yet attempted to undertake this will probably feel little sympathy for the examiners, with some justification. When multiple choice questions are used as a teaching aid, both positive and negative responses have a beneficial role. Positive answers may be expanded to underline the basic principles that have generated the question, whereas false answers allow the opportunity not only for providing the correct answer but also to broaden the discussion to bring out further teaching points.

Drs Jeswani and Morlese cover fully the curriculum in their new book in a format that parallels that of the new FRCR exam. In addition to being an educational process, reading this book should make working for the exam as enjoyable a process as possible, particularly for groups working together.

You will find the text educational, informative and accurate.

Andrew Platts
January 2005

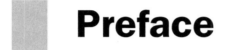

Preface

The FRCR exam is undergoing change. The new FRCR Part 1 exam was first introduced at the December 2002 sitting. Its focus has now shifted to examining the candidate's knowledge of the fundamentals of physics and radiation protection required to work safely within a radiology department.

Very few books at present are aimed at preparing the candidate for this new exam. In this book we have presented the new syllabus in a multiple choice question and answer format reflecting the format of the new exam. In addition, fundamental teaching points have been reinforced by including short answer questions.

It is hoped that this book will supplement standard texts, helping candidates not only to pass the exam but also to achieve a better and long-lasting understanding of the subject for their future careers.

Tony Jeswani
John Morlese
January 2005

About the authors

Tony Jeswani studied medicine at Guy's and St Thomas' Hospital, London. He received a first-class honours degree in radiological sciences in 1995 and was awarded the Kiri Photiou prize for his achievements. He then completed his medical degree with honours in 1998. He underwent the majority of his training in London, in particular at St George's Hospital, Tooting. He completed his MRCS (Edin) in 2002. His first book, *Viva Practice for the MRCS*, was also published in 2002. He is currently training in radiology at the Royal Free Hospital, Hampstead. He passed the FRCR Part 1 in 2002 at the first sitting of the new exam.

John Morlese received his medical degree from St George's Hospital Medical School, London in 1993. He was also awarded a degree in clinical sciences from St Mary's Hospital, London in 1992. Dr Morlese trained in clinical sciences and metabolism at the Tropical Metabolism Research Unit in Kingston, Jamaica and the Children's Nutritional Research Center, Baylor College of Medicine in Houston, Texas. He trained in general and HIV medicine at Chelsea and Westminster Hospital, London. He is currently a specialist registrar in radiology at the Royal Free Hospital, Hampstead.

This book is dedicated in memory of my father, Chuni Lal Jeswani, whom we all love and miss greatly. It is also dedicated to Madhu, Sanjaya and Kavita Jeswani and Katie Burgess for their love, support and guidance.

Tony Jeswani

I would like to dedicate this book to my father, John P Morlese, and my mother, Joyce Morlese, for their love, dedication and inspiration.

John Morlese

Section 1
Basic physics

Radiation

 Q1 The following travel at the speed of light in a vacuum. True or false?
(a) X-rays.
(b) Gamma rays.
(c) Sound waves.
(d) Radio waves.
(e) Infra-red light.

A1 (a) True – they travel at approximately 3×10^8 m/s. They do not travel much slower in air.
(b) True.
(c) False.
(d) True.
(e) True.

 Q2 With respect to x-rays describe what is meant by:
(a) photon fluence.
(b) energy fluence.
(c) intensity.

A2 (a) Photon fluence is the number of x-ray photons passing through a unit area in a particular time (T).
(b) Each x-ray photon has an individual energy. The sum of all the energies of the photons passing through a unit area in time (T) gives the total energy passing through the unit area in a particular time (T). This is called the energy fluence.
(c) The total energy passing through a unit area in unit time is the intensity, which is also known as the energy fluence rate.

(Q3) What is the relation between x-ray intensity and distance from a point source, and why is this important?

(A3) X-rays travel in straight lines. As the distance from the source increases, the intensity of radiation decreases in proportion to the square of the distance:

$$\frac{\text{New intensity}}{\text{Old intensity}} = \frac{(\text{Old distance})^2}{(\text{New distance})^2}$$

This is important as moving further away from a source of x-rays reduces the dose received by the radiologist.

(Q4) Are the following statements regarding the x-ray tube true or false?
(a) X-rays are produced when accelerated electrons hit a metal target.
(b) The energy of the accelerated electrons is converted to heat and x-rays in the proportion of 9:1.
(c) The positive cathode has a fine tungsten filament which emits electrons by thermionic emission when heated to incandescence.
(d) The anode usually has a rough and curved tungsten target.
(e) As the tube contains air, the electrons are only accelerated to half the speed of light.

(A4) (a) True.
(b) False – 99% is converted to heat and 1% to x-rays.
(c) False – the cathode is negative. The negative cathode has a fine tungsten filament which emits electrons by thermionic emission when heated to incandescence.
(d) False – it usually has a smooth and flat tungsten target.
(e) False – within the tube is a vacuum. This allows the electrons to be accelerated and thus strike the target at approximately half the speed of light.

Q5 How is the x-ray tube current affected by the filament temperature?

A5 As the filament temperature increases, there is a large increase in tube current.

Q6 How do electrons lose their energy in an x-ray tube?

A6 Each electron has kinetic energy (keV) equivalent to the kilovoltage applied between the anode and the cathode. The electrons penetrate a few millimetres into the target and then lose their energy by:
- interaction with the outer-shell electrons. This gives off heat by a large number of very small energy losses.
- interaction with either the inner-shell electron or the field of the nucleus. This results in large energy losses with the production of characteristic x-rays and bremsstrahlung, respectively.

Q7 Explain how characteristic x-rays are produced.

A7 When an electron collides with an inner-shell electron of the target atom, the inner-shell electron can be completely ejected provided the incident electron has more kinetic energy than the binding energy of the inner-shell electron. This creates a hole in the shell which can be filled by an electron from an outer shell. As this occurs, energy is released in the form of a characteristic x-ray.

Q8 Explain how bremsstrahlung x-rays are produced.

A8 If an electron approaches the nucleus of a target atom, it will be deflected. As the electron deflects and moves in a different direction, some of its energy is lost. This energy is given off as an x-ray (bremsstrahlung x-ray). In an x-ray tube, 80% or more of the x-rays are bremsstrahlung x-rays (except in special procedures, e.g. mammography).

(Q9) Answer the following questions regarding the x-ray spectra depicted in Figure 1.

X-RAY SPECTRA

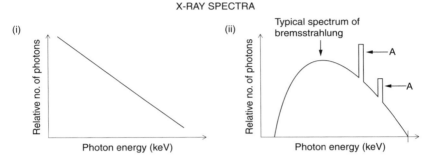

Figure 1

(a) Where might you find the x-ray spectrum depicted in (i)?
(b) Why are there no very low energy x-rays in (ii)?
(c) What do the areas labelled 'A' in (ii) represent?
(d) What is the maximum x-ray energy producible in an x-ray tube functioning at 70 kV?
(e) What does the area under the spectrum represent in real terms?

(A9) (a) The spectrum of bremsstrahlung may be found near the target nuclei.

(b) The target, the glass wall of the tube and other necessary components cause filtration of the beam. The very low energy x-rays are therefore removed.

(c) Characteristic x-ray lines.

(d) When an electron loses all of its energy on striking the target, an x-ray is produced with energy equal to the tube kV (keV). This is the maximum photon energy at this kV. In the above case, the maximum is therefore 70 keV.

(e) It is the total energy output of all x-ray photons emitted.

Atomic structure

 Q1 Name two types of ionising radiation.

A1 (a) X-rays.
(b) Gamma rays.

Q2 The following have no mass. True or false?
(a) Protons.
(b) Neutrons.
(c) Electrons.
(d) Positrons.
(e) Gamma rays.

A2 (a) False – they have a relative mass of 1.
(b) False – they have a relative mass of 1.
(c) False – they have a relative mass of 1/1840.
(d) False – they have a relative mass of 1/1840.
(e) True.

 Q3 The following have no charge. True or false?
(a) Alpha particles.
(b) Positrons.
(c) Neutrons.
(d) Gamma rays.
(e) X-rays.

A3 (a) False – they have a charge of +2.
(b) False – they have a charge of +1.
(c) True.
(d) True.
(e) True.

Q4 Where is the majority of the mass of an atom concentrated?

A4 It is concentrated within the nucleus.

Q5 What do the 'A' and 'Z' numbers of a nucleus represent?

A5 The 'A' number represents the mass number, i.e. the number of protons + neutrons in the nucleus of a particular element. The 'Z' number represents the atomic number and equals the number of protons in a particular nucleus.
Note: 'A' minus 'Z' therefore represents the number of neutrons in a particular nucleus.

Q6 In the diagram of the sodium atom given below (Figure 2) what do the letters A–E represent?

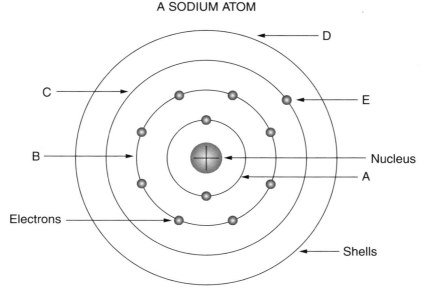

A SODIUM ATOM

Figure 2

A6   A – K-shell.
B – L -shell.
C – M-shell.
D – N-shell.
E – Valence electron (the outermost electron). The outermost shell with electrons (i.e. the valence shell) determines the chemical, optical, electrical and thermal properties of the particular element.

Q7   What is a radionuclide?

A7   It is an atom that is unstable and therefore radioactive.

Q8   What is meant by an 'ionised' atom?

A8   When an atom has had one or more of its electrons completely removed it is called an 'ionised' atom. The ionised atom is known as a positive ion.

Q9   Define the binding energy of an electron.

A9   It is the energy expended when an electron is completely removed from an atom. It is used to overcome the attracting forces of the nucleus.

Q10   How does the binding energy vary with the:
(a)   shell the electron is removed from?
(b)   element concerned?

A10   (a)   The binding energy of the K-shell is higher than that of the L-shell. In turn, the L-shell requires more energy to remove an electron than the M-shell and so on. Therefore as electrons become more distant from the nucleus, the attraction of the nucleus decreases and the energy needed to liberate them also decreases.

(b) The binding energy increases with an increase in 'Z' number (atomic number). As 'Z' increases, so does the number of protons (+1 charged particles) and therefore the attracting forces of the nucleus. Consequently, more energy is needed to liberate each electron.

(Q11) Define atomic excitation.

(A11) Atomic excitation occurs when an electron is raised from one shell to another shell which is further out. As this requires energy, the atom is said to have more energy and to be excited. When the electron 'falls' back into its original shell, the excess energy is emitted.

Interactions with matter

Q1 What are the three possible outcomes of an x-ray when it travels through matter?

A1 (a) Transmission – the x-ray is unaffected and therefore passes straight through.
(b) Absorption – all or some of the x-ray energy is given to matter.
(c) Scatter – the direction of the x-ray is altered with or without loss of energy. (Absorption + scatter is referred to as attenuation.)

Q2 What is the half-value layer (HVL) of a material?

A2 HVL is the thickness of a material required to reduce the intensity of a narrow x-ray beam to half of its original value.

Q3 How is the HVL related to the linear attenuation co-efficient (μ) of a material?

A3 $HVL = \dfrac{0.69}{\mu}$

Q4 How does the HVL vary with:
(a) increasing density of the material?
(b) increasing atomic number of the material?
(c) increasing photon energy?

(A4) (a) It decreases.
 (b) It decreases.
 (c) It increases.

(Q5) Describe the Compton scattering process.

(A5) When a photon bounces off a 'free' electron, the electron is given some energy (kinetic) and the photon is scattered, i.e. it travels in a new direction with less energy. This is the Compton scattering process. Scattering of the photons may occur in any direction. Back-scattered photons have less energy than forward-scattered photons (as more energy is imparted to the electron).

(Q6) Are the following statements true or false? If two sets of x-rays with energies of 50 keV and 150 keV are Compton scattered:
 (a) higher energy x-rays give a higher proportion of their energy to the free electrons if they are back scattered.
 (b) higher energy x-rays remain more penetrating.
 (c) recoil electrons travel further if hit by the lower energy x-rays.
 (d) lower energy x-rays produce electrons with higher kinetic energies.
 (e) the higher energy x-ray beam is softened more than the lower energy beam.

(A6) (a) True.
 (b) True.
 (c) False – higher energy x-rays make electrons recoil further than lower energy x-rays.
 (d) False – the higher x-ray energies give higher kinetic energies to the electrons.
 (e) True.

Q7 Are the following statements true or false? The Compton attenuation of an x-ray beam is related to:
(a) the atomic number of the attenuating substance.
(b) the density of the attenuating material.
(c) the energy of the x-ray beam.

A7 (a) False.
(b) True – it is proportional.
(c) True – it is inversely proportional.

Q8 Describe the process of photoelectric absorption.

A8 When an x-ray photon strikes an inner-shell (bound) electron, it can eject the electron from the atom provided it has enough energy (more than the electron's binding energy). The photon's energy (minus the energy expended in removing the electron) is given to the electron and the photon disappears completely. The ejected electron is called a photoelectron. The photoelectron leaves a hole in the inner atomic shell and an outer-shell electron can fill this hole causing the release of characteristic radiation. In the human body this radiation has low energy and is absorbed immediately.

Q9 Are the following statements true or false? Photoelectric absorption is related to:
(a) the energy of the incident x-rays.
(b) the density of the attenuating material.
(c) the atomic number of the attenuating material.

A9 (a) True – proportional to $1/E^3$ (E being the x-ray energy).
(b) True – proportional.
(c) True – proportional to Z^3 (Z being the atomic number).

Q10 As the energy of x-rays increases, the amount of photoelectric absorption decreases smoothly. True or false?

A10 False. As the energy increases, the amount of absorption decreases (proportional to $1/E^3$). However, as the energy reaches the binding energy of an electron, the amount of absorption increases. As x-ray energy further increases, absorption decreases again. This phenomenon is an exception to increasing energies causing reduced absorption and is used in choosing contrast agents at particular x-ray energies.

Q11 In the following materials which type of attenuation do diagnostic x-rays predominantly undergo?
(a) Air.
(b) Contrast media.
(c) Lead.
(d) X-ray film.
(e) Soft tissue.
(f) Bone.

A11 (a) Compton process.
(b) Photoelectric absorption.
(c) Photoelectric absorption.
(d) Photoelectric absorption.
(e) Compton process.
(f) In bone, both Compton and photoelectric processes are important.

Q12 Describe some of the properties of x-rays or gamma rays which are due to the effect of secondary electrons (recoil/photoelectrons).

A12 Ionisation causes biological tissue damage hence the dangers of ionising radiation. The excitation of some atoms makes them emit light (used to measure/detect x-rays). On x-ray films, the effect leads to the formation of an image.

 Describe why x-ray filtration is required.

 Low-energy photons are mainly absorbed by the patient. Therefore, they increase patient dose without affecting the radiographic image. They need to be removed and filters are used to do this. Filtration is inherent to the x-ray tube (x-rays are absorbed by the target, the tube housing, etc.). Additional filtration can be added in the form of aluminium. The effect on the relative number and energies of x-rays is shown below (Figure 3).

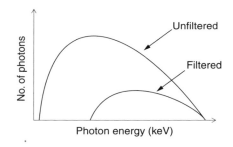

Figure 3

(Q14) What kV and filter size would be needed to produce:
(a) a 'hard' x-ray beam?
(b) a 'soft' x-ray beam?

(A14) (a) A high kV with a thick filter (x-rays with a high effective energy).
(b) A low kV with a thin filter.

Section 2
X-rays

X-ray tube

Q1 How is overheating prevented in the target of an x-ray tube?

A1 A large area of the target is used in x-ray production. This spreads out the heat produced. In addition, the exposure time can be increased. This spreads the heat over a greater period of time.

Q2 How are the following reduced?
(a) Movement blurring.
(b) Focal spot size.

A2 (a) Reducing exposure time can reduce movement blurring.
(b) Reducing the focal area of the target bombarded to produce x-rays can reduce focal spot size.

It can be seen that a trade-off exists between the above and tube heating (*see* Q1). A compromise is reached by focusing the electrons onto a small area of the target and using a rotating anode.

Q3 What is the target angle of an anode?

A3 The angle between the central ray and the anode face is called the target angle. It is shown in Figure 4.

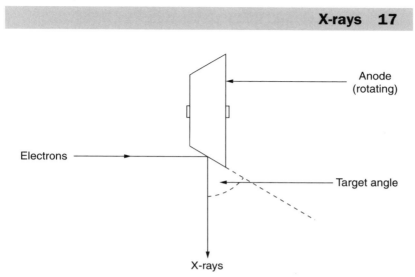

Figure 4

Usually the angle is approximately 10–20 degrees, and an x-ray tube has two filaments and two focal spots of different sizes.

(Q4) How does the target angle affect the effective focal spot size?

(A4) The smaller the target angle, the smaller the effective focal spot size (for the same actual focal spot size). In addition, the x-ray beam is narrower and a smaller field is covered.

(Q5) Name two ways of measuring the effective focal spot size.

(A5) (a) Using a star test tool (example shown in Figure 5).
(b) Using a pin-hole camera.

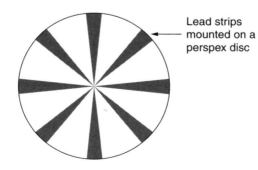

Figure 5

Q6 What is 'blooming' and when does it occur?

A6 Blooming is an increase in focal spot size. It occurs when a high tube current is used (especially if a low kV and a small focal spot are used).

Q7 Are the following statements regarding the rotating anode true or false?
(a) The anode cools by conduction and radiation of heat.
(b) The anode disc is usually 3 cm in diameter.
(c) The anode is usually made of a tungsten alloy.
(d) The anode never rotates faster than 850 rpm.

A7 (a) True – the rate of radiation increases as the anode gets hotter.
(b) False – it can be 10 cm or more.
(c) True – this has a longer life expectancy compared with just tungsten.
(d) False – it can rotate 10–20 times faster.

Q8 What is the anode heel effect?

A8 Most electrons travel a very short distance into the target before being stopped. On exiting the target, the x-rays produced are attenuated by the target itself. In Figure 6 x-ray 'B' traverses the target for a greater distance than 'A' and is therefore attenuated more. As you go from 'C' to 'B', the x-ray intensity decreases. This is the 'heel effect'. The smaller the target angle, the greater the heel effect. The amount of heel effect increases over the lifespan of the target.

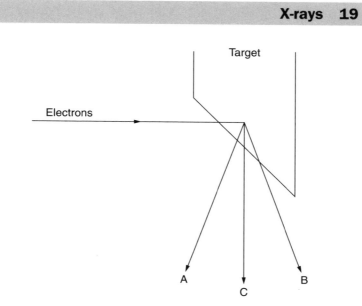

Figure 6

 The following parameters are part of the quality assurance of an x-ray tube. True or false?
(a) Focal spot size.
(b) Total filtration.
(c) Kilovoltage.
(d) X-ray output.
(e) Field definition/uniformity.

 (a) True.
(b) True.
(c) True.
(d) True.
(e) True.

Plain radiography

(Q1) Are the following statements true or false?
  (a) When taking a chest radiograph the entrance dose is about 100 times greater than the exit dose emerging from the patient.
  (b) When taking an anteroposterior (AP) abdominal radiograph the entrance dose is about 100 times greater than the exit dose emerging from the patient.
  (c) When taking an AP skull radiograph the entrance dose is about 10 times greater than the exit dose emerging from the patient.

(A1) (a) False – for a chest radiograph (posteroanterior (PA)) it is about 10 times greater.
  (b) True.
  (c) False – it is about 100 times greater.

(Q2) What effect does increasing the kV have on the entrance dose:exit dose ratio?

(A2) As the kV increases, the beam has more energy and is more penetrating, i.e. more of the incident x-rays penetrate and exit the patient. A lower entrance dose is needed to give the same exit dose. The ratio (*see* Q2) therefore decreases. In other words, by increasing kV, a lower patient dose is needed to fully expose the x-ray film.

(Q3) Are the following statements true or false?
  (a) Increasing filtration leads to a higher patient skin dose.
  (b) Increasing the x-ray focal spot to film distance leads to a higher patient skin dose.

20

A3 (a) False – increasing filtration hardens the beam and removes low energy photons which increase dose without affecting the image.

(b) False – this allows the x-rays to be spread over a larger surface area and therefore reduces skin dose. It also reduces to a lesser extent the dose to deeper structures.

Q4 Are the following statements regarding x-ray contrast true or false?

(a) Subject contrast depends on the thickness of a structure.

(b) Subject contrast depends on the difference between the linear attenuation co-efficients of the two adjacent structures from which contrast is sought.

(c) Subject contrast depends on the tissue densities of the two structures from which contrast is sought.

(d) Subject contrast depends on the atomic numbers of the two tissues from which contrast is sought.

(e) Subject contrast depends on the kV used.

A4 (a) True – the thicker the structure, the higher the contrast.

(b) True – contrast is proportional to the difference between the attenuation co-efficients of tissues.

(c) True – tissue density affects attenuation co-efficient and therefore contrast.

(d) True – atomic number affects attenuation co-efficient and therefore contrast.

(e) True – as kV increases, contrast reduces.

Q5 How do contrast media work?

A5 Contrast media are used to increase the contrast between tissues. They have high atomic numbers and absorb a lot of x-rays (at energies used in diagnostic radiology). This increases the contrast.

Q6 Are the following statements regarding magnification in an x-ray image true or false?

(a) Magnification is reduced by using a short film-to-focus distance (F).

(b) Magnification is reduced by using a large patient-to-film distance (P).

(c) Magnification is given by the formula:

$$\frac{(F + P)}{(F - P)}$$

A6 (a) False – using a long film-to-focus distance reduces magnification.

(b) False – using a small patient-to-film distance reduces magnification.

(c) False – magnification is given by the formula:

$$\frac{F}{F - P}.$$

Q7 Are the following statements regarding blurring true or false?

(a) Blurring is reduced by using a small focal spot.

(b) Blurring is reduced by using a large patient-to-film distance.

(c) Blurring is reduced by using a long film-to-focus distance.

(d) Movement blurring can be reduced with patient immobilisation techniques.

(e) Movement blurring can be reduced with shorter exposure times.

A7 (a) True – this reduces geometrical blurring.

(b) False – using a small patient-to-film distance reduces blurring.

(c) True – this also reduces distortion and magnification.

(d) True.

(e) True.

Q8 Are the following statements regarding x-ray scattering true or false?
  (a) Scattering reduces the contrast in an image.
  (b) Reducing the field size increases scatter.
  (c) Compression of the patient increases scatter.
  (d) Reducing field size increases the dose to patients.
  (e) Scatter can be reduced by using a grid.
  (f) Scatter is increased by using an air gap between the patient and the film.

A8 (a) True – scatter causes a haze over an image.
  (b) False – reducing the field size decreases scatter because there is less tissue to scatter the x-rays.
  (c) False – the amount of tissue scattering the x-rays is reduced and therefore scattering is reduced.
  (d) False.
  (e) True – anti-scatter grids reduce scatter effectively.
  (f) False – the air gap technique can be used to reduce the amount of scatter hitting the film.

Q9 The following increase the patient dose. True or false?
  (a) Compression of the patient.
  (b) Anti-scatter grids.
  (c) An air gap technique to reduce scatter.

A9 (a) False – this reduces scatter and patient dose.
  (b) True – fewer x-rays are allowed to hit the film therefore a higher dose is required to produce an adequate image.
  (c) True – this reduces scatter but causes an increase in dose and image magnification.

Q10 Draw an anti-scatter grid and describe the grid ratio.

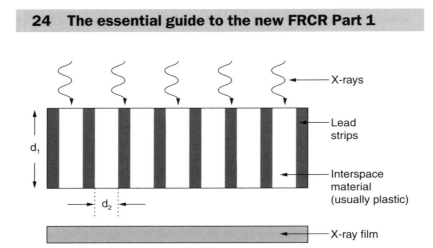

Figure 7

(A10)   The grid ratio is the depth of the interspace material (d_1) divided by the width of the interspace material (d_2) (*see* Figure 7).

(Q11)   What effect does a large grid ratio have on the efficiency of the grid to absorb scatter?

(A11)   Larger grid ratios result in more efficient absorbtion of scatter and therefore increase image contrast.

(Q12)   Give three examples of when a grid might not be used.

(A12)   Grids tend not to be used in children, when imaging 'thin' parts of the body and if there is an air gap.

(Q13)   What is a crossed grid?

(A13)   In a crossed grid two grids are superimposed with their lines at right angles. This increases scatter removal but also increases the dose required.

(Q14)   What is a 'Bucky' grid?

(A14)   This is a moving grid. It moves a short distance during the exposure perpendicular to the grid lines. This blurs out the grid lines so they are not seen on the image. The movement can be linear or circular.

X-ray tomography

(Q1) What is x-ray tomography?

(A1) It is a method of imaging a selected slice of a patient which is parallel to the film. The selected slice is imaged sharply while those slices above and below are intentionally blurred. In general, this is achieved by moving the tube and film around a stationary patient. Figure 8 shows the movement of x-ray source and film. Point 'B', which is midway between the two, forms a sharp image in the middle of the film. All other points ('A' and 'C') do not form a consistent image and are blurred.

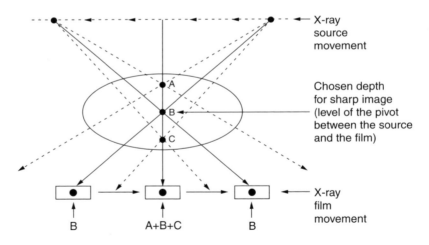

Figure 8

Q2   How does distance from the pivot plane affect blurring?

A2   The further the structure is from the pivot plane, the greater the blurring.

Q3   In radiology today, when might you use tomography?

A3   This technique is useful when conducting intravenous urography to selectively image the kidneys.

Q4   Are the following statements regarding tomography true or false?
(a)   Slice thickness is usually a few millimetres.
(b)   Contrast is usually high.
(c)   Patient dose is higher than in conventional radiography.

A4   (a)   True.
(b)   False – contrast is low since other structures are blurred across the film.
(c)   True.

Section 3
Fluoroscopy

Image intensification

(Q1)
Draw a diagram of an image intensifier and label the important components.

(A1) *See* Figure 9.

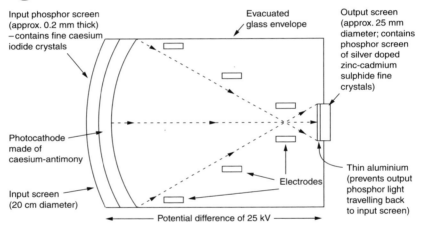

Input phosphor screen (approx. 0.2 mm thick) – contains fine caesium iodide crystals

Evacuated glass envelope

Output screen (approx. 25 mm diameter; contains phosphor screen of silver doped zinc-cadmium sulphide fine crystals)

Photocathode made of caesium-antimony

Input screen (20 cm diameter)

Electrodes

Thin aluminium (prevents output phosphor light travelling back to input screen)

Potential difference of 25 kV

Figure 9

(Q2) Describe the important steps in image intensification to produce an image.

(A2) The x-rays strike an input phosphor screen. This screen converts energy into light. The light interacts with the photocathode producing electrons that are accelerated across the potential difference between the input screen (negative) and output screen (positive). The electrons are focused onto the output screen by a number of electrodes of varying potentials that make up an 'electron lens'. The accelerated electrons strike the small output screen producing light.

Q3 Give two reasons for using caesium iodide as the input phosphor.

A3 (a) Caesium iodide is effective at absorbing x-rays at the energies used in fluoroscopy.

(b) It has fine crystals that can be packed tightly thus reducing light spread and increasing screen efficiency.

Q4 What effect does the image intensifier have on the image?

A4 The image is intensified, inverted and minified. Each x-ray photon ultimately produces approximately 400 000 light photons from the output screen.

Q5 What is the approximate overall gain for an image intensifier? What is flux gain and minification gain? What is their contribution to the overall gain?

A5 Overall gain for an image intensifier is approximately 5000 to 10 000. Flux gain is the increase in light photons produced due to higher energy accelerated electrons. This gain is approximately ×50–100. Minification gain is the increase in brightness due to a smaller image being produced from a larger input screen. It is approximately ×100 and is given by the formula:

$$\frac{\text{Input phosphor area}}{\text{Output phosphor area}}$$

Q6 When using an image intensifier, how may the edges of the image produced differ from the central image?

A6   The edges tend to be less bright, less sharp and distorted. This is due to the difficulty in controlling peripheral electrons, and is helped by using a curved input face.

Q7   What is vignetting?

A7   Vignetting means the centre of the image is brighter than the edges and is due to the electron lens system.

Q8   Define spatial resolution. How is it affected by image blurring?

A8   It is the ability to distinguish a structure from its background or the ability to see two structures as separate. Blurring worsens the resolution.

Q9   Are the following statements regarding the image intensifier true or false?
(a)   The image intensifier has a spatial resolution of 1 line pair/mm.
(b)   The majority of blurring is due to light spread in the output phosphor.
(c)   The resolution of the image is worse at the periphery than at the centre.
(d)   Image intensification can lead to 'pin cushion' distortion.
(e)   The resolution of the image is further degraded by the television system.

A9   (a)   False – it is approximately 4–5 line pairs/mm in general.
(b)   False – the majority of blurring is due to light spread in the input phosphor.
(c)   True.
(d)   True.
(e)   True.

(Q10) Are the following statements regarding contrast in an image intensifier true or false?
(a) Contrast may be reduced by backward travelling light from the output phosphor.
(b) X-rays penetrating through to the output phosphor and producing light may reduce the contrast.
(c) Glare can be caused by light scattering in the output phosphor window of the image intensifier.

(A10) (a) True.
(b) True.
(c) True – this is called veiling glare.

(Q11) Are the following statements regarding image intensifier noise true or false?
(a) Quantum noise is noticeable in fluoroscopy.
(b) In less bright areas of the image, image quality is limited by noise.
(c) Noise is representative of the statistical fluctuations in the number of x-ray photons absorbed in the input screen.
(d) A low-contrast object is less easily seen in a noise-filled image.

(A11) (a) True.
(b) True.
(c) True.
(d) True.

(Q12) Two structures may not be distinguished with an image intensifier if:
(a) the noise is too great.
(b) the contrast difference between the two structures is large.
(c) the structures are very small.
(d) the structures are very close together.
(e) higher dose rates are used.

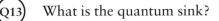

(A12)   (a)   True.

(b)   False – if the contrast difference is small, the two structures may not be distinguished.

(c)   True.

(d)   True.

(e)   False – higher dose rates reduce noise and increase the detectability of structures.

(Q13)   What is the quantum sink?

(A13)   It is the part of the system with the lowest signal-to-noise ratio and is therefore the weakest link in the imaging system.

Digital subtraction angiography (DSA) and computed tomography (CT)

Q1 Explain how images are produced in DSA.

A1 Images are taken of the area of interest before and after injection of contrast. Movement is minimised to produce the best image. The pre-contrast image, called the mask, is subtracted from the post-contrast image leaving data belonging only to the contrast-filled structures. Thus only those structures filled with contrast are seen in the subtracted image.

Q2 Are the following statements true or false? General requirements for DSA include:
- (a) a large field image intensifier.
- (b) a low-noise stable television system.
- (c) a small focal spot x-ray tube.
- (d) a low current throughout.
- (e) a manually driven contrast delivery syringe.

A2 (a) True.
(b) True.
(c) True.
(d) False – to reduce noise, the current is much higher than the usual screening current.

35

(e)   False – a motor-driven syringe is used. This is under the control of the computer doing the image subtractions.

(Q3)   Are the following statements regarding noise in DSA true or false?
(a)   The amount of noise in the subtracted image is less than in either the mask or contrast images.
(b)   The signal-to-noise ratio is improved by summing a number of mask images.
(c)   Noise in the contrast image can be reduced by summing a number of contrast images.
(d)   Patient movement makes summing multiple images more difficult.

(A3)   (a)   False – it is larger. The subtraction process reinforces the noise.
(b)   True.
(c)   True.
(d)   True.

(Q4)   Name three methods of subtraction that can be used in DSA.

(A4)   Temporal, energy and hybrid subtraction.

(Q5)   Describe the first-generation CT scanner. What was the approximate scanning time for each slice?

(A5)   The first-generation CT scanner was a translate–rotate scanner. A single beam traversed the patient and a single detector detected it (*see* Figure 10). The source and detector translated through 180 steps and then rotated through 1 degree at a time. Acquisitions were made through 360 degrees. The scan time was approximately three to five minutes per slice.

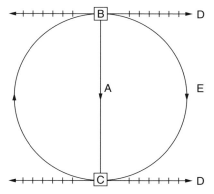

A = Single x-ray beam
B = X-ray source
C = Detector
D = Translation of equipment
E = Rotation of equipment

Figure 10

 Q6 Describe the second-generation CT scanner. What was the approximate scan time per slice?

A6 The second-generation CT scanner was a translate–rotate scanner. However, it used a fan beam of x-rays, which fell upon an array of detectors (*see* Figure 11). The source and detectors translated and then rotated through 360 degrees. Scan time was approximatelty 15–20 seconds per slice.

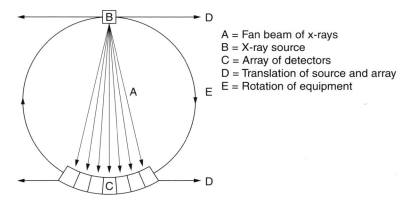

A = Fan beam of x-rays
B = X-ray source
C = Array of detectors
D = Translation of source and array
E = Rotation of equipment

Figure 11

Q7 Describe the third-generation CT scanner. What is the approximate scan time per slice? What particular artefacts is it prone to producing?

A7 The third-generation CT scanner is the commonest type of scanner used today. It is a rotate–rotate scanner. A wide fan beam of x-rays falls upon a large array of detectors which rotate continuously through 360 degrees around the patient (*see* Figure 12). Scan time is approximately 1 second per slice. The images are, however, prone to ring artefacts.

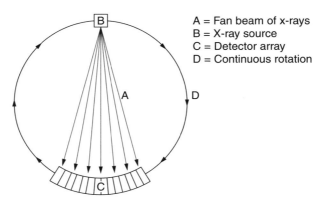

A = Fan beam of x-rays
B = X-ray source
C = Detector array
D = Continuous rotation

Figure 12

Q8 Describe the fourth-generation scanner. What is the approximate scan time per slice? What are its benefits and drawbacks compared to the third-generation scanners?

A8 In the fourth-generation scanners, the x-ray tube alone rotates through 360 degrees. The patient lies within a continuous ring of detectors which are stationary. Scan time is approximately 1 second per slice. It is easier to calibrate than the third-generation scanners and ring artefacts can be avoided. Radiation doses, however, are higher.

(Q9) What technology has made helical scanning possible?

(A9) Slip ring technology.

(Q10) Name some of the desirable features of detectors in a CT scanner.

(A10) (a) Wide dynamic range.
(b) Linearity (output proportional to x-ray intensity).
(c) Small size.
(d) High detection efficiency.
(e) Fast response.

(Q11) Name two scintillators used in CT scanner detectors.

(A11) Caesium iodide and cadmium tungstate.

(Q12) For which type of scanner are ionisation chambers useful as detectors?

(A12) Ionisation chambers are well suited to third-generation CT scanners. They are less suited to use with fourth-generation scanners.

(Q13) What is the CT/Hounsfield number for:
(a) water?
(b) air?
(c) soft tissue?

(A13) (a) 0
(b) −1000
(c) Depends on the kV used in the scanner.

Q14 How is the CT image reconstructed from the raw projection data?

 A14 The image can be reconstructed either using filtered back projection or by using a two-dimensional Fourier transformation.

 Q15 Describe what the partial volume effect is.

A15 The CT number attributed to a pixel is the average of the CT numbers of the contents of the corresponding voxel. If a voxel contains two or more different tissues, each with different attenuating abilities, the CT number is the average of the individual CT numbers. The pixel CT number, therefore, is not representative of any one of these constituents. This is called the partial volume effect and it can lead to artefacts in a CT image. A high-contrast object, e.g. a small calcification, occupying part of a voxel will increase the CT number of the corresponding pixel. It will therefore appear larger in the image.

 Q16 Name two ways of reducing the partial volume effect in a CT image.

A16 (a) Using thinner slices.
(b) Using smaller pixels.

 Q17 Describe the beam hardening effect with regard to CT scanning.

A17 As an x-ray beam penetrates a patient, lower energy x-rays are attenuated preferentially. The beam therefore becomes harder. As a result, the CT number attributed to the same kind of tissue decreases along the path of the x-ray beam. The computer compensates for this by using an algorithm. Beam hardening is reduced by using a relatively homogeneous beam, and this is produced by using a copper 'bow tie' filter on the x-ray tube.

(Q18) Name some of the benefits and problems of using a relatively high kV (120 kV) in CT scanning.

(A18) The benefits include lowering of both patient dose and beam hardening. The problems include lowering of both detector efficiency and contrast in the image. Scatter is also increased.

(Q19) Are the following statements regarding noise in CT scanning true or false?
(a) Noise can be tested by imaging a water phantom.
(b) Quantum noise is a fundamental limit of the quality of the CT image.
(c) Quantum noise reduces contrast resolution without affecting spatial resolution.
(d) Noise can be reduced by decreasing the slice thickness.
(e) Noise can be reduced by increasing the pixel size.
(f) Noise can be reduced by increasing the current used.
(g) Noise is worse when imaging thicker, i.e. obese, patients.

(A19) (a) True.
(b) True.
(c) False – it reduces the contrast resolution of small objects and reduces the spatial resolution of low-contrast objects.
(d) False – increasing slice thickness can reduce noise.
(e) True.
(f) True.
(g) True.

(Q20) Are the following statements regarding spatial resolution in CT scanning true or false?
(a) The spatial resolution with high-contrast structures is good and is determined by the noise in the image.

(b)   Spatial resolution may be tested with a bar phantom.

(c)   Spatial resolution may be affected by patient movement.

(d)   The spatial resolution with low-contrast structures is not as good as that with high-contrast structures.

(e)   A low-contrast structure has to be very small to be resolved in the image.

(f)   Perceptibility of low-contrast objects increases if the current used is increased.

 (a)   False – the spatial resolution with high-contrast structures is good and is determined by pixel size.

(b)   True.

(c)   True.

(d)   True.

(e)   False – it has to be relatively large to be resolved in the image.

(f)   True.

 Are the following statements regarding CTDI true or false?

(a)   CTDI stands for the CT detector index.

(b)   It can be measured by inserting an ionisation chamber dose meter along a phantom and then imaging a slice through it.

(c)   CTDI can be used to calculate organ doses from CT examinations.

(A21) (a)   False – it is the CT dose index.

(b)   True.

(c)   True.

(Q22) Are the following statements true or false? CT image artefacts can be caused by:

(a)   motion.

(b)   low-attenuation objects.

(c)   detector malfunction.

(d)   partial voluming.

(a) True.
(b) False – highly attenuating objects, e.g. bone, surgical clips, etc, cause CT artefacts.
(c) True – detector malfunction can cause ring artefacts in third-generation scanners.
(d) True.

 Are the following statements true or false? The advantages of spiral/helical compared with sequential CT scanning include:
(a) reduced scanning times.
(b) reduced requirement of contrast media.
(c) less partial voluming.

(a) True.
(b) True.
(c) True.

Section 4
Nuclear medicine

Radioactivity

(Q1) The following are isotopes of carbon. True or false?
(a) Carbon-13.
(b) Carbon-11.
(c) Boron-12.
(d) Carbon-14.

(A1) (a) True.
(b) True.
(c) False.
(d) True.

An isotope has the same number of protons (atomic number) but a different number of neutrons and hence a different mass number.

(Q2) What are radionuclides?

(A2) Radionuclides are unstable nuclei, which are therefore radioactive. They decay, giving off radiation until they become stable.

(Q3) Are the following statements regarding radionuclides true or false?
(a) There are many naturally occurring radionuclides.
(b) A nuclear reactor can be used to produce them.
(c) A cyclotron can be used to produce them.
(d) Radioactive fission products may be used clinically.
(e) Generators may be used to produce them.

(A3) (a) False – there are few naturally occurring radionuclides, e.g. radon and uranium.
(b) True.

(c) True.
(d) True.
(e) True.

Q4 Are the following statements regarding radionuclides true or false?
(a) Nuclear reactors produce nuclides with a neutron deficit.
(b) Nuclear reactors produce carrier-free radionuclides.
(c) A cyclotron produces nuclides with a neutron excess.
(d) Cyclotron-produced radionuclides can be carrier free.
(e) Cyclotron-produced radionuclides are typically long lived (long half-lives).
(f) A cyclotron produces nuclides by accelerating electrons to bombard stable nuclei.

A4 (a) False – nuclides with neutron excess are produced because neutrons are forced into stable nuclei.
(b) False – the radionuclides produced have the same atomic number and hence the same chemical properties as their original stable nuclide. Therefore, they cannot be separated and made carrier free.
(c) False – nuclides with neutron deficit are produced because neutrons are knocked out of stable nuclei.
(d) True – parent and daughter nuclei have different atomic numbers and can be separated to give carrier-free radionuclides.
(e) False – they are typically short lived.
(f) False – positively charged ions (e.g. alpha particles, protons) are accelerated and knock out neutrons from stable nuclei.

Q5 Are the following statements regarding radioactive decay true or false?
(a) The percentage of unstable nuclei decaying in a fixed time is predictable.
(b) One can predict which nuclei will disintegrate next.

   (c)   Disintegration of nuclei is governed by the laws of chance.

   (d)   Radioactivity is measured by the number of disintegrations in unit time.

   (e)   Activity of a radioactive sample is the number of disintegrations per hour.

   (f)   The unit of activity is the sievert.

   (g)   The human body has a natural radioactive content.

   (h)   An old unit of activity is the curie and 1 millicurie = 37 MBq (megabecquerels).

   (i)   The human body has a natural radioactive content of approximately 2 MBq.

A5
   (a)   True – hence the half-life.

   (b)   False.

   (c)   True.

   (d)   True.

   (e)   False – it is the number of disintegrations per second.

   (f)   False – it is the becquerel.

   (g)   True.

   (h)   True.

   (i)   False – it is approximately 2000 becquerels.

Q6
Are the following statements regarding the detection of beta and gamma rays true or false?

   (a)   The instruments used for detection give count rates that equal activity.

   (b)   Count rates detected are proportional to activity.

   (c)   The activity of a sample reduces by equal fractions in equal intevals of time.

A6
   (a)   False – count rates are less than activity as some of the rays miss the detector and some pass through undetected.

   (b)   True.

   (c)   True – this is known as the exponential law.

(Q7) Are the following statements regarding radioactive decay and half-life true or false?

(a) The physical half-life is the time taken for an unstable nuclide to decay to half its original activity.

(b) The physical half-life is a fixed characteristic of a radionuclide.

(c) The physical half-life is affected by heat and pressure.

(d) Activity after five half-lives is less than 1% of the original activity.

(e) Activity eventually falls to zero.

(f) Half-lives of radionuclides vary from seconds to years.

(A7) (a) True.

(b) True.

(c) False – it is unaffected by heat, pressure, chemical reaction or electricity.

(d) False – activity is approximately 3% after five half-lives.

(e) False – as decay is exponential, activity never falls to zero.

(f) True.

(Q8) What is meant by the biological half-life of a pharmaceutical?

(A8) If a pharmaceutical is injected alone, the body slowly eliminates it (metabolises/excretes it). The pharmaceutical therefore has a biological half-life, i.e. its quantity in the body falls to half its original amount in a fixed time.

(Q9) What is meant by the effective half-life of a radio-pharmaceutical?

(A9) Radionuclides are injected with pharmaceuticals. The pharmaceuticals are then considered to be labelled. Once injected, a radio-pharmaceutical reduces in activity due to decay (governed by the physical half-life) and metabolism/excretion (governed by the biological half-life). Taking both of these processes into account, an effective half-life can be calculated for the radionuclide in the body using the formula given below:

$$\frac{1}{\text{Effective half-life}} = \frac{1}{\text{Biological half-life}} + \frac{1}{\text{Physical half-life}}$$

Therefore, the effective half-life is always shorter than the biological or physical half-life. The effective half-life varies with different radio-pharmaceuticals and from person to person.

Radio-pharmaceuticals

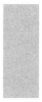

 Q1 Are the following statements true or false? Desirable properties of a radionuclide for imaging include:

(a) a very short half-life.

(b) emission of many different energy gamma rays.

(c) easy attachment to pharmaceuticals at room temperature.

(d) emission of 20 keV gamma rays.

(e) emission of gamma rays and no beta or alpha particles.

(f) being readily available/producible on site.

(g) decay to a stable daughter.

(h) being able to form a stable product with a pharmaceutical both *in vitro* and *in vivo*.

(i) forming a low toxicity radio-pharmaceutical.

A1 (a) False – if the half-life is too short, the nuclide will have decayed massively prior to administration. In general, a desirable half-life is a few hours.

(b) False – mono-energy gamma rays are ideal so scatter can be reduced by energy discrimination with the pulse height analyser.

(c) True.

(d) False – ideally 150 keV gamma rays should be used. At this energy, the gamma rays have enough energy to exit the patient but can also be collimated and detected. In general, gamma rays in the range 50–300 keV are acceptable.

(e) True.

(f) True.

(g) True.

51

(h) True
(i) True.

(Q2) Are the following statements regarding the properties of metastable technetium true or false?
(a) It emits gamma rays with an energy of 80 keV.
(b) It is a pure gamma emitter.
(c) It has a half-life of six hours.
(d) It is supplied in a generator shielded with aluminium.
(e) Sterile saline is used to wash it off an alumina exchange column on which molybdenum has been adsorbed.
(f) In the generator, technetium is washed off as sodium pertechnetate.
(g) Elution of technetium from the generator takes a few hours.
(h) Technetium generators are replaced monthly.
(i) Fulfils many of the desirable criteria described above and is thus used for the majority of radionuclide imaging.

(A2) (a) False – gamma rays with an energy of 140 keV are produced. This is ideal energy for collimation and detection.
(b) True.
(c) True.
(d) False – it is supplied in a generator but this is shielded with lead.
(e) True.
(f) True.
(g) False – elution takes a few minutes.
(h) False – the generator is replaced weekly.
(i) True.

(Q3) Are the following statements regarding the usage and labelling of technetium true or false?
(a) Technetium can be used for thyroid imaging.
(b) Technetium can be used for salivary gland imaging.

(c) Technetium can be used for cerebral blood flow imaging.

(d) Technetium can be labelled to DMSA for renal studies.

(e) Technetium can be labelled to HIDA for biliary studies.

(f) Technetium can be used for lung ventilation studies.

 A3

(a) True.
(b) True.
(c) True.
(d) True.
(e) True.
(f) True.

Q4 Are the following statements regarding thallium-201 true or false?

(a) It is produced in a cyclotron.
(b) It emits 130 keV photons when it decays by electron capture.
(c) It can be used for myocardial perfusion studies.
(d) It has a half-life of six hours.

A4

(a) True.
(b) False – it emits 80 keV photons.
(c) True.
(d) False – it has a half-life of 73 hours.

Q5 Are the following statements regarding indium-111 true or false?

(a) It is produced in a cyclotron.
(b) It has a half-life of six hours.
(c) It emits 173 keV and 247 keV gamma rays.
(d) It can be used for localising abscesses.

A5

(a) True.
(b) False – it has a half-life of 67 hours.
(c) True.
(d) True.

(Q6)   Are the following statements regarding metastable krypton-81 true or false?
(a)   It is produced in a cyclotron.
(b)   It has a half-life of 13 minutes.
(c)   It emits 100 keV x-rays.
(d)   The generator is eluted with saline and then the krypton gas is extracted.
(e)   It can be used in ventilation/perfusion scanning.
(f)   It can be stored and used over one week before a new generator is needed.

(A6)   (a)   False – it is produced in a generator.
(b)   False – the half-life is 13 seconds.
(c)   False – 190 keV gamma rays are emitted.
(d)   False – the generator is eluted with air which the patient then inhales.
(e)   True.
(f)   False – its parent has a short half-life of four to five hours.

(Q7)   Are the following statements true or false? Quality control (QC) of radio-pharmaceuticals includes assessing:
(a)   sterility.
(b)   radionuclide purity.
(c)   chemical purity.
(d)   radiochemical purity.

(A7)   (a)   True.
(b)   True.
(c)   True.
(d)   True.

Gamma imaging

Q1   Describe how gamma imaging produces an image.

A1   A patient is given a radio-pharmaceutical (orally, intra-venously or via inhalation) which concentrates in an area of interest. The radionuclide gives off gamma rays which are collected and recorded by a gamma camera. An image is produced on a monitor delineating the distribution of the nuclide within the body.

Q2   Draw a schematic diagram of a gamma camera labelling all the important components.

A2   *See* Figure 13.

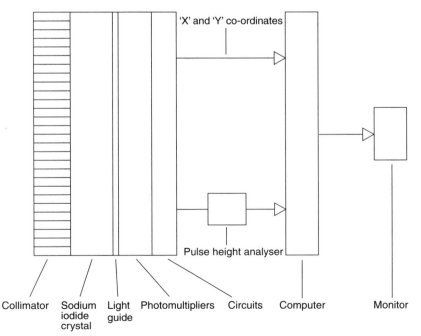

Figure 13

Q3   Are the following statements regarding the collimator in a gamma camera true or false?
(a)   It is made of a lead disc.
(b)   It is approximately 25 cm thick.
(c)   It is up to 20 mm in diameter.
(d)   It has many hexagonal or circular holes in it.
(e)   The holes are usually 2.5 cm in diameter.
(f)   There are approximately one million holes in it.
(g)   The holes are separated by septa which are 3 mm thick.
(h)   It is used to absorb most gamma rays not parallel to the collimator.

A3   (a)   True.
(b)   False – it is 25 mm thick.
(c)   False – it is up to approximately 400 mm in diameter.
(d)   True.
(e)   False – they are usually 2.5 mm in diameter.
(f)   False – there are approximately 20 000 holes.
(g)   False – they are approximately 0.3 mm thick.
(h)   True.

Q4   Explain how a collimator is able to locate the position of a radioactive source.

A4   *See* Figure 14. Each hole accepts gamma rays from a narrow channel. These impinge on the crystal and produce an image (A and B). Gamma rays that are not parallel to the holes are absorbed by the lead septa and do not produce an image (C and D). Some gamma rays are scattered (E) and can enter through the collimator. However, these rays have less energy than non-scattered gamma rays and can be excluded from the image by the pulse height analyser.

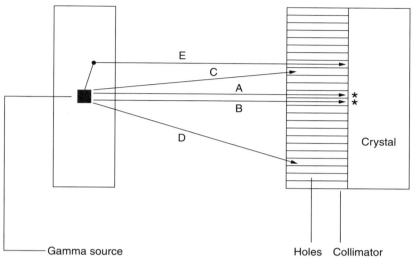

Figure 14

Q5 Are the following statements regarding the gamma camera crystal true or false?
(a) It is made up of millions of small crystals.
(b) It typically has a diameter of 50 mm and a thickness of 100 mm.
(c) It is typically made of caesium iodide activated with thallium.
(d) It absorbs approximately 99% of gamma rays produced by technetium.
(e) It is fragile and easily damaged by moisture and light.
(f) Each absorbed gamma photon produces approximately 5000 light photons.
(g) The light produced is then recorded by photomultipliers.

A5 (a) False – it is one large crystal.
(b) False – the diameter is usually about 500 mm with a thickness of approximately 10–12 mm.
(c) False – it is typically made of sodium iodide activated with thallium.
(d) False – approximately 90% are absorbed.

(e) True.
(f) True.
(g) True.

Q6 Are the following statements regarding the photomultipliers in a gamma camera true or false?
(a) There are usually five in a loosely packed array.
(b) Each photomultiplier is an evacuated glass envelope with a photocathode coated with a light absorber which emits photoelectrons.
(c) Each light photon produces 10 photoelectrons.
(d) Photoelectrons are accelerated towards dynodes. On impinging upon the dynodes, more electrons are produced.
(e) With the multiplication of electrons in the photo-multipliers, each flash of light is able to produce a measurable voltage.

A6 (a) False – there are up to 90 in a tightly packed array.
(b) True.
(c) False – 5–10 light photons produce one electron.
(d) True.
(e) True.

Q7 How does information from the photomultipliers locate the origin/position of the light flash from the crystal?

A7 A pulse arithmetic is used (position logic) to locate the position of the light flash. The light pulse produces electrical pulses of different sizes in a number of photomultipliers. The largest pulse is formed in the photomultiplier nearest to the collimator hole through which the gamma ray passed. Smaller pulses are formed in adjacent photomultipliers.

The pulse arithmetic circuit combines the information from the photomultiplier tubes and gives X and Y co-ordinates for the gamma ray. In addition, a value for the photon energy of the incident gamma ray is obtained. Scattered photons and those undergoing Compton interactions in the crystal prior to being absorbed are detected as having less energy.

Q8 Draw a pulse height spectrum. Describe its different components.

A8 *See* Figure 15.

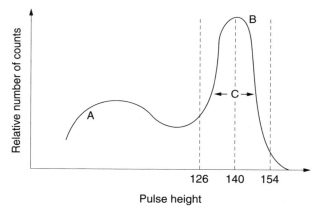

Figure 15

A – Compton tail. These are low energy pulses mostly from gamma rays undergoing Compton scatter in the patient or crystal.

B – Photopeak. These are pulses from gamma rays completely absorbed without any Compton scatter.

C – Full width at half maximum (FWHM).

Q9 What does a pulse height analyser do?

A9 This rejects pulses with too low or too high energies (outside the dashed lines in Figure 15). It lets through pulses of ±10% of the photopeak. However, some of the scattered gamma rays only lose a little energy and are consequently accepted thus degrading the image.

 Q10 Name four types of collimator that can be used for gamma imaging. Which is the commonest?

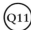 **A10** (a) Parallel hole – this is the commonest. The field of view and sensitivity are the same at all distances from its face.
(b) Divergent hole.
(c) Convergent hole.
(d) Pinhole.

Q11 Under what circumstances might you use a:
(a) divergent hole collimator?
(b) convergent hole collimator?
(c) pinhole collimator?

 A11 (a) When imaging a large field of view with a small crystal, e.g. with a mobile gamma camera.
(b) When image magnification is required. The field of view is reduced. This can be useful when imaging children.
(c) When a magnified inverted image is desired. It is useful for small superficial organs, such as the thyroid.

Q12 What are some of the problems associated with divergent and convergent hole collimators?

A12 (a) They cause geometrical distortion.
(b) Different depths within the patient are magnified differently.
(c) The field of view and sensitivity vary with distance.

Q13 What is the sensitivity of a collimator? What factors affect it?

 A13 The sensitivity is the percentage of gamma rays passing through the holes. Less than 1% of gamma rays actually pass through. The collimator can have a higher sensitivity if there are:
(a) more holes.
(b) wider holes.
(c) shorter holes.

Higher sensitivity means less radioactivity needs to be used and therefore a smaller patient dose.

Q14 Explain what is meant by the spatial resolution of a collimator.

A14 *See* Figure 16. 'R' represents the spatial resolution of the collimator. It is larger (i.e. worse spatial resolution) the further you are from the face of the collimator.

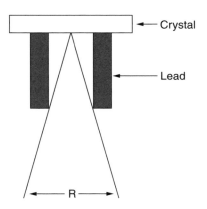

Figure 16

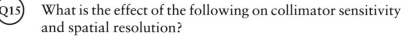

Q15 What is the effect of the following on collimator sensitivity and spatial resolution?
(a) Wide collimator holes.
(b) Short collimator holes.

A15 (a) Increases sensitivity but decreases spatial resolution.
(b) Increases sensitivity but decreases spatial resolution.

Therefore a compromise between spatial resolution and sensitivity needs to be reached.

Q16 How are the following assessed for gamma imaging?
(a) Uniformity of field.
(b) Spatial resolution.
(c) Linearity of the system (lack of distortion).
(d) Sensitivity.

A16 (a) Using a flood field phantom.
(b) By imaging a line source, which gives the line spread function.
(c) By imaging a line source.
(d) Using a flood field phantom.

Q17 Are the following statements regarding spatial resolution true or false?
(a) Intrinsic resolution is the spatial resolution of the camera with the collimator but no patient present.
(b) Intrinsic resolution can be improved by using a thicker crystal.
(c) System resolution is the resolution of the camera with the collimator and patient present.
(d) Resolution is better in obese patients.
(e) Resolution is better if the radioactive source is further away from the collimator.

(a) False – it is the camera resolution without a collimator or a patient.

(b) False – it can be improved by using a thinner crystal, which reduces sensitivity.

(c) True.

(d) False.

(e) False – the opposite is true.

Patient dose in gamma imaging

 Q1 Are the following statements regarding absorbed dose to an organ true or false?
- (a) Absorbed dose to an organ increases in proportion to activity administered to the patient.
- (b) Absorbed dose to an organ increases in proportion to the fraction of activity taken up by the organ.
- (c) Absorbed dose to an organ increases in proportion to the effective half-life of the activity in the organ.
- (d) Absorbed dose to an organ decreases exponentially with increasing energy of radiation emitted.

 A1
- (a) True.
- (b) True.
- (c) True.
- (d) False – it increases in proportion.

Q2 Are the following statements regarding the effective dose true or false?
- (a) Dose increases if more images are taken.
- (b) All tissues in the body receive equal dose.
- (c) In general, the patient's brain gets the highest dose.
- (d) An average dose to the body as a whole can be calculated.
- (e) Effective dose is measured in milligrays cm^2.

 A2
- (a) False – dose is unaffected by the number of images taken.
- (b) False – different tissues receive different doses.

(c) False – in general, the target organ and the organs of excretion get the highest dose.

(d) True – this is the effective dose.

(e) False – it is measured in sieverts.

 Q3 How can the patient dose be minimised once the test has started?

A3 The dose can be minimised if the patient drinks lots of water and empties their bladder regularly. This reduces pelvic and gonadal dose.

Single-photon emission computed tomography (SPECT) and positron emission tomography (PET)

Q1 Describe how a SPECT image is produced.

A1 A gamma camera with a parallel-hole collimator rotates around a patient on a couch. After every 6 degrees it stops and acquires data for approximately 30 seconds. It continues to do this for 360 degrees around the patient. The data sets produced are synthesised into a transverse image by filtered back projection.

Q2 Are the following statements regarding SPECT true or false?
(a) The images are severely photon limited.
(b) Noise is low.
(c) Spatial resolution is better than that of conventional gamma imaging.
(d) Three-dimensional images may be produced.

A2 (a) True.
(b) False – due to limited counts at each angle, the noise is high.

(c) False – it is worse.
(d) True.

  Q3 Are the following statements regarding PET true or false?
Positive beta emitters include:
(a) Carbon-12.
(b) Nitrogen-13.
(c) Oxygen-16.
(d) Oxygen-17.
(e) Fluorine-18.

A3 (a) False – carbon-11 gives off positrons.
(b) True.
(c) False.
(d) False – oxygen-15 gives off positrons.
(e) True.

Q4 Are the following statements regarding PET true or false?
(a) Nitrogen-13 is produced in a generator.
(b) Carbon-11 has a half-life of 80 minutes.
(c) Positrons travel approximately 5 mm in a patient prior
to annihilation.
(d) Annihilation produces two 511 keV photons in prac-
tically opposite directions.

A4 (a) False – it is produced in a cyclotron.
(b) False – it has a half-life of 20 minutes.
(c) False – positrons travel less than 1 mm prior to annihilation.
(d) True.

Q5 Are the following statements regarding a positron camera
true or false?
(a) The camera is composed of a large number of photomultiplier tubes coupled to caesium iodide detectors.
(b) Only impulses that produce simultaneous pulses are
detected.

(c)   The bismuth germanate detectors are more sensitive than a conventional gamma camera.

A5   (a)   False – the photomultiplier tubes are coupled to bismuth germanate detectors.
(b)   True.
(c)   True.

Q6   Are the following statements regarding PET imaging true or false?
(a)   Dose to the patient is higher than in routine gamma imaging.
(b)   It has a better resolution than SPECT.
(c)   Gallium-68 can be used for imaging.
(d)   Gallium-68 is produced in a cyclotron.

A6   (a)   False – the dose is much the same.
(b)   True.
(c)   True.
(d)   False – it is produced in a generator.

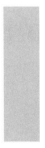

Section 5
Radiation protection

Radiation protection and regulations

Q1 Are the following statements regarding the deterministic effects of x-rays true or false?
- (a) They are characterised by a threshold effect.
- (b) They result generally from cell death.
- (c) They include skin erythema, hair loss, sterility and cataracts.
- (d) Typical features of acute radiation syndrome include nausea, vomiting, diarrhoea and anorexia.
- (e) They are irreversible.

A1
- (a) True.
- (b) True.
- (c) True.
- (d) True.
- (e) False.

The severity of an effect depends on the radiation dose and occurs once the threshold has been exceeded.

Q2 Are the following statements regarding the stochastic effects of x-rays true or false?
- (a) The severity of radiation-induced effects is independent of radiation dose.
- (b) Radiation dose affects the probability of a stochastic effect occurring.
- (c) Stochastic effects have a threshold effect.
- (d) They are independent of sex and age at exposure.
- (e) Radiation protection has no effect on stochastic radiation risk.

A2 (a) ⎫ True. The probability of an effect occurring is depen-
         ⎬ dent on the radiation dose. These effects include can-
    (b) ⎭ cer and genetic effects.
    (c) False.
    (d) False.
    (e) False – the aim of radiation protection is to reduce the
         risk of stochastic effects of radiation.

Q3 Are the following statements true or false?
    (a) All tissues have similar susceptibility to radiation-
         induced malignancy.
    (b) Cancer risks are higher for adults than children.
    (c) Radiation induces malignant and not benign tumours.
    (d) Radiation induces solid tumours earlier than leu-
         kaemia.
    (e) Radiation-induced thyroid cancer is more common in
         men than in women.

A3 (a) False – there is great variability in the sensitivity of
         different tissues to radiation.
    (b) False – cancer risks are greater in children.
    (c) False.
    (d) False – leukaemia occurs earlier after an exposure
         than solid tumours.
    (e) False.

Q4 Are the following statements true or false?
    (a) The dose limits for employees under 18 years of age
         are typically higher than for older workers.
    (b) The effective dose limit for a worker over 18 years of
         age is similar to the effective dose from a barium meal
         examination.
    (c) The effect of radiation *in utero* is the same regardless
         of the stage of exposure.
    (d) Microcephaly is a recognised effect of radiation ex-
         posure *in utero*.

(e)   Mental retardation tends to occur with early *in utero*
        exposure.

(A4)   (a)   False.
        (b)   True.
        (c)   False.
        (d)   True.
        (e)   True.

Table 1   Annual dose limits defined in the Ionising Radiations
Regulations 1999 (IRR 1999)

	>18 years	<18 years	Others
Dose limits for the whole body (mSv)	20	6	1
Dose limits for individual organs and tissues (mSv)	500	150	50
Dose limits for the lens of the eye (mSv)	150	50	15

The risk to the fetus is dependent on the gestational age.
The fetus is most vulnerable to congenital abnormalities
during the first trimester. Microcephaly and mental retardation occur with exposure in late first trimester and second
trimester, respectively. Intrauterine death tends to occur
with very early exposures and malignancies in later pregnancy.

(Q5)   Are the following statements regarding radiation units true
        or false?
        (a)   Exposure is measured in coulombs/kg.
        (b)   Absorbed dose is the quantity of ionisation produced
               in a given mass of air by a given quantity of radiation.
        (c)   Absorbed dose is the amount of energy imparted per
               unit mass to a medium by the incident radiation.
        (d)   The weighting factor for x-rays and gamma rays is 1.
        (e)   Equivalent dose is the overall biological effectiveness
               of a given radiation dose.

A5 (a) True.
(b) False – absorbed dose is the amount of energy imparted per unit mass to a medium by the incident radiation. It is measured in grays (J/kg).
(c) True.
(d) True.
(e) True.

Q6 Are the following statements true or false?
(a) Annual average radiation exposure is approximately 2.5 mSv.
(b) On average, approximately 15% of the total annual radiation exposure dose is due to medical exposure.
(c) Radon and thoron are important contributors to annual average radiation exposure.
(d) Food and drink and cosmic radiation contribute similar amounts of radiation to the annual average radiation exposure.
(e) There is a geographical variation in the annual average radiation exposure.

A6 (a) True.
(b) True.
(c) True.
(d) True.
(e) True.

Q7 Are the following statements regarding radiation-induced malignancies true or false?
(a) Stomach cancer has a higher death rate per mSv per million than liver cancer.
(b) Leukaemia has a higher death rate per mSv per million than thyroid cancer.
(c) Osteosarcoma is an example of a radiation-induced malignancy.
(d) Breast cancer can be induced by screening mammography.

    (e)   They are examples of the deterministic effects of radiation.

(A7)   (a)   True.
    (b)   True.
    (c)   True.
    (d)   True.
    (e)   False – malignancies are examples of stochastic effects.

(Q8)   Are the following statements regarding the sources of x-ray exposure true or false?
    (a)   Palpating the patient with a lead glove in the primary beam does not affect dose to the patient.
    (b)   Leakage of radiation at a distance of 1 m from the focus should not exceed 1 µSv.
    (c)   Lead equivalent of 2.5 mm is typical for image intensifier housing.
    (d)   The primary beam cannot be altered to decrease the dose to the patient.
    (e)   Scattered radiation contributes 1% of the total patient dose in fluoroscopy.

(A8)   (a)   False – palpating the patient with a lead glove increases the patient dose.
    (b)   False – leakage of radiation at a distance of 1 m from focus should not exceed 1 mSv.
    (c)   True.
    (d)   False – the primary beam can be affected by filtration and collimation to decrease patient dose.
    (e)   True – scattered radiation contributes 1% of total patient dose in fluoroscopy.

(Q9)   Are the following statements regarding radiation exposure during pregnancy true or false?
    (a)   Few deterministic or stochastic effects occur in live-born children exposed to radiation during the first three weeks of life.

(b) High-dose examinations such as barium enemas or computed tomography of the abdomen/pelvis can be performed within the first 10 days of pregnancy.
(c) The approximate risk of inducing a cancer in a child is 1 in 1000.
(d) Radiation exposure during pregnancy can lead to early death.
(e) Shields have minimal effects on protecting the fetus.

A9 (a) True.
(b) True.
(c) True.
(d) True.
(e) False.

Q10 Are the following statements regarding attempts to decrease patient dose true or false?
(a) Increasing the distance from the patient by 50% decreases the dose to the operator by a factor of 4.
(b) The preset timer typically has a maximum of 20 minutes.
(c) If a part of the body is not in the primary beam, a protective barrier is unnecessary.
(d) Protective lead aprons mainly protect against the primary beam.
(e) Gloves of 0.35 mm lead equivalent protect against the primary beam.

A10 (a) False – the inverse square law is important in reducing patient dose and dose to operator.
(b) False – there is no upper limit; the preset exposure timer is usually set at 5 minutes.
(c) False.
(d) False – protective lead aprons protect against scattered x-rays and absorbs 90% of these rays.
(e) False.

Q11 Are the following statements true or false?
(a) X-ray rooms do not require special construction.
(b) All x-ray room walls are lined with lead.
(c) Regarding shielding, 1 mm of lead is equivalent to 120 mm of barium plaster.
(d) X-ray rooms are designed and constructed to decrease the exposure to workers and the public to less than 0.1 mSv per week.
(e) The design of x-ray walls is primarily to stop scattered radiation.

A11 (a) False – x-ray rooms require special construction so as to minimise the exposure to workers and passers-by in adjacent rooms or corridors.
(b) False.
(c) False – 1 mm of lead is equivalent to 12 mm of barium plaster and 120 mm of concrete in its ability to absorb x-rays.
(d) True.
(e) True.

Q12 Are the following statements regarding film badges true or false?
(a) They are double coated.
(b) They are not affected by changes in ambient humidity.
(c) They cannot distinguish different types of radiation.
(d) The minimum dose detectable is 0.15 mSv.
(e) Calibration is unnecessary.

A12 (a) False.
(b) False.
(c) False.
(d) True.
(e) False.

This is the most commonly used method of personal dosimetry. Film badges have a range of 0.15–1000 mSv and can differentiate between types of radiation exposure. They consist of a fast and slow emulsion and are calibrated with a gamma ray source.

Q13 Are the following statements regarding film badges true or false?
(a) They consist of fast and slow emulsions.
(b) They are typically assessed six monthly.
(c) They are assessed by measuring the density of blackening of the film.
(d) They consists of two filters.
(e) Neutron exposure cannot be assessed.

A13 (a) True.
(b) False.
(c) True.
(d) False – they contain three filters typically consisting of plastic, aluminium and tin.
(e) False.

Film badges are worn for a month, and then they are processed under controlled conditions. The densities are assessed.

Q14 Are the following statements regarding film badge dosimetry true or false?
(a) They typically have high and low gamma emulsions.
(b) Different types of radiation can be differentiated.
(c) Control films are used during processing.
(d) Lithium fluoride is used.
(e) Fading of the latent image is a problem.

A14 (a) True.
(b) True.
(c) True.
(d) False – lithium fluoride is used in thermoluminescent dosimeters (TLDs).
(e) True.

Q15 Are the following statements regarding thermoluminescent dosimeters (TLDs) true or false?
(a) Silver bromide is used to trap excited electrons in electron traps.
(b) Lithium fluoride is the preferred phosphor.
(c) They have a memory for trapped electrons.
(d) They are assessed by measuring the density of blackening of the film contained within them.
(e) They can be assessed using a Geiger–Müller counter.

A15 (a) False.
(b) True.
(c) True.
(d) False.
(e) False.

TLDs use lithium fluoride as the phosphor which absorbs x- or gamma rays. The radiation causes electrons to be elevated into electron traps. These excited electrons remain in the traps. The TLDs are read by heating to 300 °C in a light-sealed container and light is emitted as the excited electrons return to their ground state. The amount of light emitted is proportional to the exposure.

Q16 Are the following statements regarding TLDs true or false?
(a) They are heated to greater than 300 °C to trap electrons.
(b) Heating results in emission of light from the phosphor.
(c) The amount of light emitted is inversely proportional to the dose of radiation absorbed by the phosphor.
(d) Calibration is unnecessary as the phosphor has a long-term memory.
(e) They have to be discarded after a single use.

A16 (a) False.
(b) True.
(c) False.

(d)   False – calibration is necessary with a gamma ray source.
(e)   False – TLDs have a high initial cost but are re-usable.

Q17   Are the following statements regarding TLDs true or false?
(a)   TLDs commonly use lithium fluoride.
(b)   When heated, electrons enter the conduction band and emit light.
(c)   The amount of light emitted is no longer proportional to the dose of radiation absorbed above 5 mSv.
(d)   Different filters are used including plastic and lead.
(e)   Lithium and fluorine have low atomic numbers, making lithium fluoride a good tissue equivalent.

A17   (a)   True.
(b)   True.
(c)   False.
(d)   False.
(e)   True.

Q18   Are the following statements regarding electron personal dosimeters (EPDs) true or false?
(a)   They are very sensitive especially at low photon energies (<40 keV).
(b)   They are less sensitive than TLDs.
(c)   They require manual assessment to produce an accurate read-out.
(d)   They can be particularly useful for pregnant workers.
(e)   They are single-use devices.

A18   (a)   False.
(b)   False.
(c)   False.
(d)   True.
(e)   False.

EPDs generate a real-time read-out. They are poorly sensitive to low energy photons, but the sensitivity is greater than TLDs. EPDs are useful for pregnant workers as the time and quantity of the exposure can be monitored closely. EPDs are re-usable devices.

Q19   Are the following statements regarding personal dose systems true or false?
(a)   TLDs provide an immediate read-out of dose data.
(b)   EPDs have a non-linear response to dose.
(c)   EPDs provide a real-time read-out of dose data.
(d)   TLDs are not useful in distinguishing radioactive contamination.
(e)   TLDs are re-usable.

A19   (a)   False.
(b)   False – EPDs have a linear response to dose.
(c)   True.
(d)   True.
(e)   True.

Q20   Are the following statements regarding personal dosimetry true or false?
(a)   Film badges have an effective dose range of approximately 0.2–1000 mSv.
(b)   Film badges produce a permanent record.
(c)   Protective gloves have a minimum lead equivalent of 0.25 mm.
(d)   The dose limits for employees under 18 years of age are typically higher than for older workers.
(e)   The effective dose limit for a worker over 18 years of age is similar to the effective dose received from a barium meal examination.

A20   (a)   True.
(b)   True.
(c)   True.
(d)   False.
(e)   True.

Radiation detection

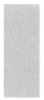

Q1 Are the following statements regarding Geiger–Müller tubes true or false?
  (a) They can differentiate between different types of radiation.
  (b) They can differentiate between different energies of same radiation.
  (c) They are good at detecting beta particles.
  (d) They are better than ionisation chambers at detecting gamma rays.
  (e) Dead time is not a significant problem.

A1 (a) False – Geiger–Müller tubes detect ionisation produced but do not differentiate between types.
  (b) False.
  (c) False – they are inefficient at detecting high-energy beta particles and have a low detection efficiency for gamma rays.
  (d) True.
  (e) False – the dead time is 100 μs and is a period when tube cannot produce further pulses.

Q2 Are the following statements regarding Geiger–Müller tubes true or false?
  (a) They contain an inert gas alone.
  (b) They use a mica window to detect alpha and beta particles.
  (c) The typical voltages used differ depending on whether alcohol or halogen is used in the tube.
  (d) A lead cathode is typically used.
  (e) A vacuum is used within the tube.

(A2)   (a) False – Geiger–Müller tubes contain an inert gas with either a halogen gas or alcohol at low pressures in the ratio 9:1.
(b) True.
(c) True – the voltage applied across the tube depends on whether a halogen gas or alcohol is added and is higher for alcohol.
(d) True.
(e) False.

(Q3)   Are the following statements regarding scintillation tubes true or false?
(a) Scintillation tubes are used for the quantitative measurement of radiation.
(b) They emit light when exposed to radiation.
(c) The light emitted is detected by photomultiplier tubes (PMTs).
(d) The output voltage from the PMTs is inversely proportional to the amount of energy absorbed by the scintillator substance.
(e) Calcium tungstate can be used in a scintillation tube.

(A3)   (a) True.
(b) True.
(c) True.
(d) True.
(e) True.

(Q4)   Are the following statements regarding radiation protection principles true or false?
(a) The basis of justification for a radiation exposure is that the benefit outweighs the risk to the patient.
(b) The effective dose should be as low as reasonably practicable for workers and visitors.
(c) Legal limits have been prescribed for exposures relating to workers and members of the public.

(d) Dose limits are designed to reduce the probability of stochastic effects and eliminate deterministic effects.

(e) A radiographer's annual radiation dose regularly exceeds the dose limit for a member of the public.

(A4) (a) True.
(b) True.
(c) True.
(d) True.
(e) False – a radiographer's annual radiation dose is usually much less than the public dose limits.

(Q5) Are the following statements regarding radiation quantities true or false?

(a) Equivalent dose is measured in milligrays (mGy).
(b) Equivalent dose is the effective dose multiplied by radiation weighting factors relating to the radiation used.
(c) Equivalent dose is used to compare doses from different radiology techniques applied to a particular organ.
(d) Absorbed dose multiplied by a radiation weighting factor gives the equivalent dose.
(e) Equivalent and effective doses are interchangeable.

(A5) (a) False – the absorbed dose is measured in grays (Gy), the equivalent dose and effective dose are measured in sieverts (Sv).
(b) False – equivalent dose is equal to absorbed dose multiplied by the radiation weighting factor (biological effectiveness of radiation dose).
(c) True.
(d) True.
(e) False.

(Q6) Are the following statements regarding effective dose true or false?

(a) It is measured in millisieverts (mSv).

(b)   For alpha particles, the absorbed dose is numerically greater than the equivalent dose.

(c)   For x-rays and gamma rays, the absorbed dose is often numerically equal to the equivalent dose.

(d)   The effective dose is measured in J/kg.

(e)   Radiation weighting factors are measured in units of joules (J).

A6   (a)   True.
(b)   False.
(c)   True.
(d)   True.
(e)   False.

Effective dose is the sum of the different organ doses multiplied by a weighting factor for each organ. The weighting factors have no units.

Q7   Are the following statements regarding ionising radiation true or false?

(a)   It exerts its biological effects on organs by ion production and energy deposition that damage molecules.

(b)   Alpha particles produce the same amount of biological damage for the same amount of energy deposited as gamma rays.

(c) LD_{50} is the dose of radiation that would kill 50% of the population.

(d)   It affects bone marrow cells the most.

(e)   It affects the liver and breast tissue to greatly differing extents.

A7   (a)   True.
(b)   False.
(c)   True.
(d)   True.
(e)   True.

The radiation weighting factor for alpha particles is 20 and for x-rays and gamma rays it is 1.

Q8 Are the following statements regarding diagnostic refer-
ence levels (DRLs) true or false?
(a) They need to be established locally for all radiological
examinations.
(b) DRLs should be reviewed annually.
(c) For computed tomography (CT), a radiation-induced
cancer risk of up to 1 in 1000 per examination can be
seen.
(d) All exposures exceeding the DRL should be reported
to the Department of Health.
(e) If the DRL is exceeded the examination must be stopped
immediately.

A8 (a) False – DRLs are generally derived from nationally
obtained data unless the radiological department has
special reasons for having different exposures, e.g. age
of equipment.
(b) True.
(c) True.
(d) False.
(e) False – the examination does not need to be stopped
at that moment but an investigation should be performed thereafter to determine the cause.

Q9 Are the following statements regarding effective dose true
or false?
(a) The typical dose for an intravenous urogram (IVU) is
similar to that of a barium meal.
(b) The typical dose for an abdominal radiograph (AXR)
is similar to 1000 chest radiographs (CXR).
(c) The typical dose for a skull radiograph is 0.15 mSv.
(d) Typical doses for a barium enema and CT abdomen
scan are similar.
(e) The typical dose for a Tc^{99m} MDP bone scan is 5 mSv.

A9 (a) True.
(b) False.

(c) True.
(d) True.
(e) True.

Table 2 Effective dose in various investigations

Investigation	Effective dose (mSv)
CXR	0.02
AXR	1.5
Skull radiograph	0.15
IVU	5.0
Barium meal	5.0
Barium enema	9.0
CT abdomen	9.0
Tc^{99m} MDP bone scan	5.0

 Are the following statements regarding factors affecting the exposure time true or false?
(a) The exposure time is increased by increasing the kV.
(b) The exposure time is increased by decreasing the kV.
(c) Exposure time can be decreased by using a smaller focal spot.
(d) Use of a three-phase generator decreases exposure time.
(e) Use of a full wave single-phase generator decreases exposure time.

A10 (a) False.
(b) True.
(c) False.
(d) True.
(e) True.

The exposure time is reduced by increasing the kV and using a larger focal spot, three-phase generator or full wave rectification.

(Q11) Are the following statements true or false? Regarding organ
dose, the tissue weighting factors for the following tissues
are as given below.
(a) Bone marrow – 0.2.
(b) Bladder – 0.2.
(c) Skin – 0.12.
(d) Liver – 0.05.
(e) Breast – 0.05.

(A11) (a) True.
(b) False – it is 0.05.
(c) False – it is 0.01.
(d) True.
(e) True.

(Q12) Are the following statements true or false?
(a) A supervised area is an area where the annual dose is
likely to exceed 3/10 but be less than 6/10 of the
annual dose limit.
(b) LD_{50} (Lethal dose to 50%) is typically 5 Gy.
(c) The risk of developing a fatal cancer is 1 in 10 000 per
mSv.
(d) The maximum risk from radiation to a fetus is between 8 and 16 weeks *in utero* during organogenesis.
(e) Body aprons generally have a lead equivalent of 0.25–
0.35 mm.

(A12) (a) False – a supervised area is an area where the annual
dose is likely to exceed 1/10 but be less than 3/10 of the
annual dose limit.
(b) True.
(c) True.
(d) True.
(e) True.

Q13 The following represent the average effective dose for the associated common radiological procedure. True or false?
(a) Barium enema – 9.0 mSv.
(b) IVU – 5.0 mSv.
(c) Lumbar spine radiograph – 2 mSv.
(d) CT abdomen – 1 mSv.
(e) Thallium-67 cardiac scan – 1 mSv.

A13 (a) True.
(b) True.
(c) True.
(d) False.
(e) False.

The effective dose for a CT abdomen is approximately 9.0 mSv and for a Thallium-67 cardiac scan is 25 mSv.

Q14 Are the following statements regarding radiation protection true or false? Dose-saving techniques include using:
(a) a smaller field size.
(b) grids.
(c) a large focus-to-object distance.
(d) shields.
(e) digital radiography.

A14 (a) True.
(b) False – grids reduce scatter and increase contrast but increase patient dose.
(c) True.
(d) True.
(e) True.

Q15 The following represent the typical effective doses for the procedures expressed as the equivalent number of CXRs. True or false?
(a) Tc^{99m} bone scan – 200.
(b) CT head – 1000.

(c) CT pelvis – 500.
(d) Barium meal – 200.
(e) AXR – 35

(A15) (a) True.
(b) False – the effective dose for a CT head is 5 mSv (250 CXRs).
(c) True.
(d) True.
(e) True.

(Q16) Are the following statements regarding the dose from various studies true or false?
(a) Barium enemas contribute more to the UK collective radiation dose than CXRs.
(b) Dental radiographs are performed more frequently than lower limb radiographs.
(c) Mammography contributes much more to the UK collective radiation dose than brain CT scans.
(d) CT scans as a group contribute most to the UK collective radiation dose.
(e) Barium enemas and abdominal CT scans, as individual examinations, contribute most to the UK collective radiation dose.

(A16) (a) True.
(b) True.
(c) False – although more mammographic investigations are performed, CT brain examinations contribute more to the UK collective radiation dose.
(d) True.
(e) True.

Legislation

Q1 Are the following statements true or false?
- (a) The Health and Safety Executive enforces the Ionising Radiations Regulations 1999 (IRR 1999).
- (b) IRR 1999 deals principally with radiation exposures to workers.
- (c) Local rules are a legal document.
- (d) Radiation protection advisers (RPAs) are often superintendent radiographers.
- (e) Diagnostic radiology workers typically receive radiation doses greater than the public dose limit.

A1
- (a) True.
- (b) True.
- (c) True.
- (d) False – radiation protection supervisors (RPSs) are typically superintendent radiographers. RPAs are often medical physicists.
- (e) False – in general, diagnostic radiology workers typically receive radiation doses much less than the public dose limit.

Q2 Are the following statements regarding the Ionising Radiations (Medical Exposure) Regulations 2000 (IR(ME)R 2000) true or false?
- (a) The referrer is responsible for providing enough clinical information to allow justification of the medical exposure.
- (b) Chiropractors and osteopaths may be referrers.
- (c) Radiographers may be referrers.
- (d) A practitioner is a registered health professional entitled to take responsibility for a medical exposure.
- (e) Practitioners are usually radiologists.

90

(A2)   (a)   True.
    (b)   True.
    (c)   True.
    (d)   True.
    (e)   True.

(Q3)   Are the following statements regarding IR(ME)R 2000 true or false?
    (a)   An operator is any person who can carry out any practical part of the medical exposure.
    (b)   Radiographers are usually the operators.
    (c)   Radiographers cannot authorise a medical radiation exposure.
    (d)   Justification of a medical radiation exposure involves the assessment of risk versus benefit.
    (e)   The over-riding principle is to keep the radiation dose as low as reasonably practicable.

(A3)   (a)   True.
    (b)   True.
    (c)   False.
    (d)   True.
    (e)   True.

(Q4)   Are the following statements true or false?
    (a)   The role of the RPA is to advise the employer on the application of the IRR 1999.
    (b)   The RPS supervises work in areas where local rules are required.
    (c)   The employer is responsible for exposure reduction, training, risk assessment and quality assurance.
    (d)   A classified worker is an employee likely to receive an effective dose >6 mSv or 6/10 employee equivalent dose.
    (e)   Records of radiation exposure are kept for 50 years or until age 75.

A4   (a)   True.
    (b)   True.
    (c)   True.
    (d)   False – a classified worker is an employee likely to receive an effective dose >6 mSv or >3/10 employee equivalent dose.
    (e)   True.

Q5   Are the following statements regarding legislation true or false?
    (a)   Radiopharmacists and cardiologists are likely to be classified workers.
    (b)   The Health and Safety Executive records doses of classified workers.
    (c)   A controlled area is where a person is likely to be exposed to >6 mSv or 3/10 of equivalent dose.
    (d)   A supervised area is where a person is likely to be exposed to >1 mSv or 1/10 of equivalent dose.
    (e)   For women of reproductive capacity the equivalent dose to the abdomen is <13 mSv in three months.

A5   (a)   True.
    (b)   True.
    (c)   True.
    (d)   True.
    (e)   True.

Q6   Are the following statements regarding IR(ME)R 2000 true or false?
    (a)   Ionising radiation is defined as the transfer of energy in the form of particles or electromagnetic waves of wavelength of ≤ 100 nm or a frequency of $\geq 3 \times 10^{15}$ Hz capable of producing ions.
    (b)   Clinical audit is not a part of the regulations.
    (c)   Practitioner means a registered medical practitioner, dental practitioner or other health professional.

(d) Operator means a registered health professional who is entitled to refer individuals to a practitioner for medical exposure.

(e) Incorporates the European Union directive, Council Directive 97/43/Euratom.

(A6) (a) True.

(b) False.

(c) True.

(d) False – referrer means a registered medical practitioner, dental practitioner or other health professional who is entitled to refer individuals for medical exposure to a practitioner.

(e) True.

(Q7) Are the following statements regarding IR(ME)R true or false?

(a) IR(ME)R only applies to NHS hospitals.

(b) The regulations do not apply to medical exposures made as part of occupational heath surveillance.

(c) The regulations do not apply to medical exposures made as part of research programmes.

(d) The regulations are enforceable under the Health and Safety at Work Act 1974.

(e) Documentation of patient radiation dose is unnecessary as it is recorded on the radiograph.

(A7) (a) False.

(b) False.

(c) False.

(d) True.

(e) False – documentation of patient exposure dose is mandatory and should be kept for at least 6 years.

Q8 Are the following statements regarding IRR 1999 true or false?

(a) For trainees aged less than 18 years, the equivalent dose limit for the hands, forearms, feet and ankles shall be 150 mSv in a year.

(b) For workers over 18 years of age, the equivalent dose limit for the lens of the eye is 50 mSv in a calendar year.

(c) Decisions about who can be a practitioner are taken at the local level.

(d) IRR includes provisions for handling radioactive materials.

(e) IRR includes provisions that cover Ministry of Defence related exposures.

A8 (a) True.
(b) False.
(c) True.
(d) True.
(e) True.

Q9 Are the following statements regarding IR(ME)R true or false?

(a) The operator is responsible for justifying the medical exposure.

(b) The operator is responsible for the practical aspects of the medical exposure.

(c) It is not possible for an individual to act concurrently as an employer, referrer, practitioner and operator.

(d) The regulations state the dose limits for students less than 18 years of age.

(e) Outside workers are not covered by the regulations.

 A9 (a) False.
(b) True.
(c) False.
(d) False.
(e) True.

The practitioner is responsible for the justification of a medical exposure. However, the operator can authorise an exposure using guidelines produced by the practitioner as it is often not possible for the practitioner to justify all exposures. Provisions for dose limits for students ≤18 years and outside workers are made in the IRR (1999). The practitioner is responsible for the justification of a medical exposure.

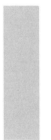

Section 6
Specialised plain radiography

Mammography, xeroradiography, tomography and high kV radiography

 Q1 Are the following statements regarding mammography true or false?
(a) The mean glandular dose (MGD) is approximately 0.8 mGy.
(b) Use of a grid increases the MGD.
(c) A typical radiation-induced breast cancer fatality rate is five per million women examined.
(d) Grids typically improve contrast by a factor of 2.
(e) Grids typically increase radiation dose by a factor of 2–3.

A1 (a) True.
(b) True.
(c) True.
(d) True.
(e) True.

 Q2 Are the following statements regarding mammography true or false?
(a) Focal spots sizes of >0.5 mm are used to maximise geometric unsharpness.
(b) Large focal spots require longer exposure times.
(c) Magnification is best achieved with a large focal spot.
(d) Magnification is best achieved with a small focal spot.
(e) A smaller focal spot produces less blurring than a larger focal spot.

A2 (a) False.
(b) False.
(c) False.
(d) True.
(e) True.

Typically small focal spots are used (approx. 0.3 mm). Increasing the focal spot size will result in shorter exposure times. Magnification is best achieved with smaller focal spots.

Q3 Are the following statements true or false? Typical features of mammography include:
(a) a small focal spot.
(b) use of an air gap technique.
(c) better resolution than plain radiographs.
(d) better signal-to-noise ratio than plain radiographs.
(e) better geometric unsharpness than plain radiographs.

A3 (a) True.
(b) True.
(c) True.
(d) True.
(e) True.

Q4 Are the following statements regarding mammographic technique true or false?
(a) The typical beam energy is 20 keV.
(b) Tungsten is used most frequently as the target material.
(c) Molybdenum produces characteristic x-rays suitable for mammography.
(d) The mean energy of characteristic x-rays produced by rhodium is greater than that produced by molybdenum.
(e) Higher energy x-rays decrease subject contrast.

A4 (a) True.
(b) False – tungsten can be used as the target material for large breasts, however, molybdenum is most frequently used in mammography.

(c)   True.
(d)   True.
(e)   True.

Q5   Are the following statements regarding mammographic technique true or false?
(a)   The anode heel effect is always detrimental.
(b)   Rhodium windows are used.
(c)   Molybdenum filters are used to remove low-energy photons.
(d)   Automatic exposure control is not typically utilised in mammography.
(e)   A higher film gamma is used in mammography than for a chest radiograph.

A5   (a)   False – placing the cathode side of the tube towards the patient where the breast is thicker uses the anode heel effect.
(b)   False – a beryllium window is used.
(c)   True.
(d)   False.
(e)   True.

Q6   Are the following statements regarding compression in mammography true or false?
(a)   It is achieved using molybdenum paddles.
(b)   It increases patient dose.
(c)   It increases sharpness and decreases scatter.
(d)   Compressed breasts are typically 4–8 cm thick.
(e)   It spreads the breast tissue allowing easier detection of a mass.

A6   (a)   False – compression is performed with radiolucent paddles.
(b)   False – compression leads to reduced patient dose.
(c)   True – compression leads to greater sharpness and reduced scatter.
(d)   True.
(e)   True.

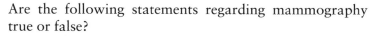

Q7 Are the following statements regarding mammography true or false?
(a) Grids are not used in mammography.
(b) Grids decrease patient dose.
(c) Scatter increases with increasing breast thickness.
(d) Grids reduce scatter and therefore improve image quality.
(e) Grids remove a greater proportion of the primary beam than of the scattered x-rays.

A7 (a) False.
(b) False.
(c) True.
(d) True.
(e) False.

Grids are used to increase contrast. They remove proportionately more scatter than primary beam. This is a function of the grid ratio (4:1). Grids increase patient dose.

Q8 Are the following statements regarding mammography standards true or false?
(a) Mammography has an invasive cancer detection rate of 3.6 per 1000 women aged 50–53 years having their first screen.
(b) It reduces the case fatality rate by 100%.
(c) It uses increased magnification.
(d) It uses a molybdenum anode.
(e) It uses typical x-ray tube peak voltages of 80–100 kV.

A8 (a) True.
(b) False – typically mammography should reduce case fatality rate by approximately 40%.
(c) True.
(d) True.
(e) False – the x-ray tube peak voltages are 20–30 kV.

Are the following statements regarding mammography true or false?

(a) The effective dose is typically 0.5–1 mSv.

(b) It produces one new breast cancer per million women screened.

(c) It has a spatial resolution of 5 line pairs/mm.

(d) It uses a wide air gap technique.

(e) Calcium tungstate can be used as a target material for smaller breasts.

(a) True.

(b) True.

(c) True.

(d) True.

(e) False – calcium tungstate can be used as a target material for larger breasts.

Table 3   Summary of mammographic technique

Mo characteristic radiation	17.9–19.5 keV
Focal spot	0.3 mm
Beryllium window	Minimal filtration
Air gap	Increased $\approx$2 times
Grid	Moving
Resolution	5 line pairs/mm
Effective dose	0.5–1 mSv
Radiation risk	1/1 000 000 women screened

Are the following statements regarding xeroradiography true or false?

(a) It produces increased edge enhancement.

(b) It has broad exposure latitude compared with film-screens.

(c) It produces increased fine structure contrast.

(d) It has the same patient exposure dose per exposure as film-screen.

(e) It has fast development times.

(a) True.
(b) True.
(c) True.
(d) False.
(e) True.

The main advantages of xeroradiography are increased edge contrast, wide latitude and increased resolution.

Q11   Are the following statements regarding xeroradiography true or false?
(a) It is prone to artefacts.
(b) X-rays reaching the plate cause the plate to lose charge.
(c) The soft tissue detail is reduced by overlying structures.
(d) The plates are fragile.
(e) The plates are re-usable.

A11   (a) True.
(b) True.
(c) True.
(d) True.
(e) True.

The main disadvantages of xeroradiography are artefacts, increased patient dose and the requirement for careful handling.

Q12   Are the following statements regarding xeroradiography true or false?
(a) Selenium-coated aluminium x-ray plates are used.
(b) Molybdenum targets are used.
(c) Uses large focal spots of >0.5 mm.
(d) The plates are re-usable.
(e) It requires similar processing equipment to film-screen combinations.

(a) True.
(b) False.

(c)   False.
(d)   True.
(e)   True.

Table 4   Summary of xeroradiographic technique

Detector	Amorphous selenium
Focal spot	0.3 mm
Anode	Tungsten
X-ray tube	45 kV
Filtration	1–2 mm
Spatial resolution	15 line pairs/mm

Q13   Are the following statements regarding xeroradiography true or false?
(a)   Typical filtration values are equivalent to 1–2 mm of aluminium.
(b)   It produces edge enhancement and wide latitude.
(c)   It gives higher mean glandular doses than for screen-film mammography.
(d)   By using a high kV, it enables visualisation of thick dense breast tissue that would otherwise not be seen with low kV screen-film combinations.
(e)   It represents the commonest form of imaging in breast radiology.

A13   (a)   True.
(b)   True.
(c)   True.
(d)   True.
(e)   False – film-screen mammography is most widely used and xeroradiography is declining in use.

Q14   Are the following statements regarding tomography true or false?
(a)   It is used for tissues with low contrast.
(b)   It utilises blurring.
(c)   Phantom images are a potential problem.

(d) The thickness of the slice is inversely proportional to the tomographic angle.

(e) Patient dose is lower than with conventional plain radiography.

A14
(a) True.
(b) True.
(c) True.
(d) True.
(e) True.

Q15 Are the following statements regarding tomography true or false?
(a) The x-ray tube and film cassette move in the same direction.
(b) Zonography uses a slice thickness large enough to include a whole organ.
(c) Tomographic movements are always linear.
(d) The fulcrum determines the level of tomographic slice.
(e) Digital radiography has removed the need for plain tomography.

A15
(a) False – in linear tomography there is simultaneous but opposite movement of the anode and film cassette.
(b) True.
(c) False – there are different patterns of movement including elliptical, circular and hypocycloidal.
(d) True.
(e) False.

Q16 Are the following statements regarding tomography true or false?
(a) The slice thickness is increased by increasing the angle of swing.
(b) The slice thickness is increased by increasing the film–focus distance (FFD).

(c)   Linear tomography typically produces thinner slices than zonography.

(d)   Linear tomography typically uses a larger tomographic angle than zonography.

(e)   It is often used for intravenous urography.

 A16
(a)   False.
(b)   True.
(c)   True.
(d)   True.
(e)   True.

Increasing the angle of swing and decreasing the focus–film distance reduce the slice thickness. Zonography uses a smaller tomographic angle and produces a thicker slice hence the whole of an organ can be included in the slice.

Q17   Are the following statements true or false?
(a)   Compared with conventional radiography subject contrast is reduced in high kV radiography.

(b)   Compared with conventional radiography skin dose is reduced in high kV radiography.

(c)   Compared with conventional radiography exposure time is reduced in high kV radiography.

(d)   High kV radiography can be used for plain chest radiography.

(e)   High kV radiography has no effect on patient dose.

A17
(a)   True.
(b)   True.
(c)   True.
(d)   True.
(e)   False.

Table 5   Features of high kV radiography

Heat loading	Reduced
Exposure time	Reduced
Skin dose	Reduced
Subject contrast	Reduced
Scattered radiation	Increased
Air gap	Used

Are the following statements regarding spatial resolution true or false?

(a)   Xeroradiography typically has a spatial resolution of 12–20 line pairs/mm.

(b)   Film-screen combinations typically have a spatial resolution of 10–15 line pairs/mm.

(c)   Spatial resolution of single and double emulsion screens is similar.

(d)   It is usually expressed in line pairs/mm.

(e)   Film alone has a better spatial resolution than film-screen combinations.

(a)   True.

(b)   False.

(c)   False – spatial resolution is decreased in double emulsion screens compared with single screens.

(d)   True.

(e)   True – film-screen combinations are associated with increased unsharpness.

Table 6   Spatial resolution values

Detector	Line pairs/mm
No screen	100
Slow screen	10
Fast screen	5
Xeroradiography	15
Mammography	5
Digital subtraction angiography	2

Film-screen combinations

Q1 Are the following statements regarding the film base true or false?
(a) It is usually made of polyester.
(b) It contains silver halide.
(c) It provides support for the emulsion.
(d) It typically has a thickness of 150 μm.
(e) It has no effect on image quality.

A1 (a) True.
(b) False.
(c) True.
(d) True.
(e) False.

The film base provides support for the emulsion and typically measures 150 μm. The film base can increase parallax in double screen-films.

Q2 Are the following statements regarding the film emulsion true or false?
(a) It contains only silver bromide grains and gelatin.
(b) The gelatin enables even dispersion of silver halides.
(c) It consists of approximately 90% silver iodide and 10% silver bromide.
(d) Allylthiourea is added to aid sensitisation.
(e) Reducing the proportion of silver iodide decreases the sensitivity of the film.

108

(a) False.
(b) True.
(c) False.
(d) True.
(e) True.

The emulsion is typically 10 μm thick and contains 90% silver bromide and 10% silver iodide dispersed in gelatin.

Q3 Are the following statements regarding intensifying screens true or false?
(a) They improve image contrast at the expense of increasing patient radiation dose.
(b) They shorten exposure times.
(c) They improve spatial resolution.
(d) Mammography is best performed with double intensifying screens.
(e) They reduce motion artefact.

A3 (a) False.
(b) True.
(c) False.
(d) False.
(e) True.

Intensifying screens increase film contrast and film unsharpness while decreasing exposure times and patient dose.

Q4 Are the following statements regarding intensification screens true or false?
(a) Gadolinium oxysulphide and lanthanum oxybromide are examples of rare earth screens.
(b) Screen unsharpness is due to diffusion of light in the phosphor.
(c) Parallax occurs only with double emulsion films.
(d) Double emulsion screens double the speed and contrast of the film-screen combination.
(e) Slow screens have an intensification factor of 100.

(A4) (a) True.
(b) True.
(c) True.
(d) True.
(e) False.

The main disadvantages of intensification screens are (i) screen unsharpness, which is due to diffusion of light in the phosphor layer and (ii) parallax, which is due to x-rays that expose different areas of the film in double emulsion films. Double emulsion screens double the speed and contrast of the film-screen combination. Slow screens typically have an intensification factor (IF) of 35 and rapid screens have an IF of 100.

(Q5) Are the following statements regarding intensifying screens true or false?
(a) Each intensifying screen consists of a base and a phosphor layer only.
(b) Rare earth screens have a conversion efficiency of 20%.
(c) Calcium tungstate has a conversion efficiency of 20%.
(d) Rare earth screens contain an element with a high atomic number.
(e) Rare earth screens amplify the effect of incident x-rays by producing light which exposes the film.

(A5) (a) False – the two layers are bound by resin.
(b) True.
(c) False.
(d) True.
(e) True.

Table 7 Typical values for different types of intensification screen

Factor	Calcium tungstate	Rare earth screen
Absorption	30%	60%
Conversion efficiency	5%	20%
Screen efficiency	50%	50%
Intensification factor	Increased	Increased

Q6 Are the following statements regarding intensification factors true or false?
  (a) The intensification factor can be increased by the use of titanium oxide between the base and the phosphor.
  (b) If the intensification factor is increased, it will decrease patient dose.
  (c) Intensification factor increases with increasing photon keV.
  (d) They can be increased by using a thicker screen layer.
  (e) They can be increased by using larger crystals in the screen layer.

A6 (a) True.
  (b) True.
  (c) True.
  (d) True.
  (e) True.

Q7 Are the following statements regarding intensification factors true or false?
  (a) They are calculated as the exposure required with a screen divided by the exposure without a screen.
  (b) The higher the intensification factor the faster the screen and the lower the patient dose.
  (c) They are inversely proportional to the thickness of the phosphor layer.
  (d) They are directly proportional to conversion efficiency and absorption.
  (e) They are unrelated to the phosphor crystal size.

A7 (a) False – calculated as exposure required without the screen divided by exposure with the screen.
  (b) True.
  (c) False.
  (d) True.
  (e) False.

The intensification factor increases with x-ray beam keV, the screen thickness and phosphor crystal size.

(Q8) Are the following statements true or false? Rare earth screens when compared with calcium tungstate screens have a:
(a) higher conversion efficiency.
(b) higher absorption efficiency.
(c) higher k-edge.
(d) higher speed.
(e) maximum light output at approximately 430 nm.

(A8) (a) True.
(b) True.
(c) False – they have a lower k-edge.
(d) True.
(e) False – calcium tungstate screens have a maximum light output at approximately 430 nm. The maximum light output for gadolinium oxysulphide occurs at 545 nm.

(Q9) Are the following statements regarding film-screen combinations true or false? For one x-ray photon absorbed by the phosphor:
(a) 60 000 light photons are produced by the phosphor.
(b) 600 light photons are produced by the phosphor.
(c) 300 light photons reach the film.
(d) 300 latent images are produced.
(e) three latent images are produced.

(A9) (a) False – one x-ray photon absorbed by the phosphor produces 600 light photons.
(b) True.
(c) True.
(d) False – 300 light photons reach the film and produce three latent images in the emulsion.
(e) True.

Q10 Are the following statements regarding film-screen quality assurance true or false?
(a) This involves measuring the film density after development.
(b) This involves the use of a sensitometer.
(c) A wide variation of densities is permissible.
(d) A sensitometer can be used to measure fog level, speed and film gamma.
(e) It is a necessary requirement to minimise patient dose.

A10 (a) True.
(b) True.
(c) False – a narrow variation of densities is permissible, typically ±10–15%.
(d) True.
(e) True.

Q11 Are the following statements regarding the x-ray film true or false?
(a) The front of the x-ray film cassette is made of carbon or aluminium.
(b) The back of the x-ray film cassette is made of lead to reduce backscatter.
(c) The film cassette is designed to reduce scatter.
(d) Double emulsion films are used for all plain radiography.
(e) Quality control of film cassettes is performed annually.

A11 (a) True – this decreases attenuation of the primary beam (low atomic number elements) and lowers patient dose.
(b) True.
(c) True.
(d) False.
(e) False.

Q12 Are the following statements regarding film-screen combinations true or false?
(a) The sensitivity of the film must match the light emission from the screen.
(b) Orthochromatic film sensitive to green light can be used with gadolinium and lanthanum screens.
(c) Rare earth screens use a lower kV.
(d) Typical values for intensification with a film-screen combination are 30–100.
(e) A screen phosphor layer can absorb x-rays better than emulsion.

A12 (a) True.
(b) True.
(c) True.
(d) True.
(e) True.

Q13 Are the following statements true or false? Calcium tungstate screens have the following properties:
(a) absorption efficiency – 60%.
(b) conversion efficiency – 5%.
(c) screen efficiency greater than rare earth screens.
(d) typical screen efficiency – 50%.
(e) increased intensification factor with increasing crystal size.

A13 (a) False.
(b) True.
(c) False.
(d) True.
(e) True.

Calcium tungstate screens have an absorption efficiency, conversion efficiency and screen efficiency of 30%, 5% and 50%, respectively. The corresponding values for rare earth screens are 60%, 20% and 50%, respectively.

Q14 Are the following statements true or false? The intensification factor of a film-screen is increased by:
(a) increasing the kV of the primary beam.
(b) increasing the phosphor crystal size.
(c) increasing the screen thickness.
(d) using a double intensification screen.
(e) using a rare earth screen instead of a calcium tungstate screen with the same thickness.

A14 (a) True.
(b) True.
(c) True.
(d) True.
(e) True.

Q15 Are the following statements regarding rare earth screens (compared with calcium tungstate) true or false?
(a) Smaller focal spots may be used with rare earth screens.
(b) They are faster than calcium tungstate screens.
(c) They have increased quantum mottle.
(d) They produce less distortion.
(e) They produce less blurring.

A15 (a) True.
(b) True.
(c) True.
(d) True.
(e) True.

Q16 Are the following statements regarding film-screen combinations true or false?
(a) Most x-rays are absorbed by the photoelectric effect.
(b) Single emulsion film is used in digital radiography.
(c) The conversion efficiency is the quantity of x-rays absorbed by the screen divided by the quantity of light emitted.

(d) Intensifying screens should contain an element with a high atomic number to increase x-ray absorption.

(e) They improve image contrast.

 (a) True.

(b) True.

(c) False – conversion efficiency is the quantity of light produced by the screen for each x-ray absorbed.

(d) True.

(e) True.

Q17 Are the following statements true or false? Increasing the screen thickness of the film-screen combination:

(a) increases the film speed.

(b) decreases the spatial resolution.

(c) decreases patient dose.

(d) increases noise.

(e) decreases exposure times.

 (a) True.

(b) True.

(c) True.

(d) False – it has no effect on noise but worsens resolution.

(e) True.

Q18 Are the following statements true or false? Increasing the conversion efficiency of a film-screen combination:

(a) increases quantum mottle.

(b) decreases spatial resolution.

(c) increases film-screen speed.

(d) decreases patient dose.

(e) generally has no effect on spatial resolution.

A18 (a) True.

(b) False.

(c) True.

(d) True.

(e) True.

Increasing the conversion efficiency reduces the number of x-rays required to make the image and hence increases noise but has no net effect on spatial resolution.

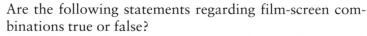 Are the following statements regarding film-screen combinations true or false?
(a) When a light photon is absorbed by the film crystal, electrons migrate to the sensitivity speck.
(b) Mobile silver ions are attracted to sensitivity specks to be neutralised.
(c) A latent image is formed by silver ions at the sensitivity speck.
(d) A latent image is permanent but not visible to the naked eye.
(e) The image becomes permanent once developed.

(A19) (a) True.
(b) True.
(c) True.
(d) False.
(e) False.

Latent images are not permanent and only become permanent when developed, fixed and washed.

 Are the following statements regarding x-ray noise true or false?
(a) Noise is inversely proportional to the number of x-rays.
(b) Increased noise reduces contrast.
(c) Increasing the number of x-ray photons absorbed increases the signal-to-noise ratio.
(d) Intensifying screens increase noise.
(e) Slow or detail screens require a higher x-ray exposure and give a high signal-to-noise ratio.

(A20) (a) True.
(b) True.
(c) True.

(d) True.
(e) True.

(Q21) Are the following statements regarding the film-screen combination in mammography true or false?
(a) Rare earth intensifying screens are used.
(b) Intensifying screens are applied to only one surface of the film.
(c) The absorption efficiency of the rare earth screens used in mammography is approximately 50%.
(d) Mammography films have high gradients and low film latitudes.
(e) Quality control for mammography is the same as that for standard plain radiography.

(A21) (a) True.
(b) True.
(c) True.
(d) True.
(e) False – quality control for mammography is more rigorous. Quality control of the automatic exposure control and processor/sensitometer is carried out daily and of the x-ray output weekly.

(Q22) Are the following statements regarding quality assurance true or false?
(a) Daily checks include beam alignment and focal spot size.
(b) The film density should be checked daily.
(c) Film density can be assessed with a 'step wedge' image.
(d) The focal spot is assessed annually with a star test tool.
(e) The x-ray tube output should be checked annually.

(A22) (a) False – these are assessed annually.
(b) True.
(c) True.
(d) True.
(e) False – x-ray tube output is checked every three months.

Q23   Are the following statements regarding quality assurance in plain radiography true or false?
(a)   Tube kilovoltage should be within 5% of the stated value.
(b)   Tube kilovoltage has to be measured directly.
(c)   Tube kilovoltage is measured using copper plates and a photodiode.
(d)   A penetrameter can display the nature of the kV waveform.
(e)   Total filtration of the x-ray beam is not usually assessed.

A23   (a)   True.
(b)   False.
(c)   True.
(d)   True.
(e)   False.

The tube kilovoltage is assessed by measuring the kV and the half-value layer.

Characteristic curve of x-ray films

 Q1 Are the following statements regarding film fog true or false?
(a) It is the density of unexposed film.
(b) Film fog reduces contrast.
(c) It is due to the film base absorbing light.
(d) It is due to storage and poor handling.
(e) It is due to the formation of a latent image during manufacture.

A1 (a) True – film fog is the optical density of processed but unexposed film.
(b) True.
(c) True.
(d) True.
(e) True.

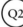 **Q2** Are the following statements regarding the characteristics of x-ray films true or false?
(a) The typical diagnostic range is 0.25–2.
(b) The unexposed film density is usually 0.
(c) Base plus fog density is approximately 0.15.
(d) They are unaffected by development parameters.
(e) Base and fog density are similar for most film-screen combinations.

A2 (a) True.
(b) False – the fog level contributes to the film density and therefore the film density cannot be zero. Hence developed but unexposed film has a density of approximately 0.15.

(c) True.

(d) False – development properties are important factors that affect the characteristic curve of a film.

(e) True.

 Q3 Are the following statements regarding the characteristic curve true or false?

(a) It is a plot of film density against exposure.

(b) It is not possible for x-ray exposure to reduce film density.

(c) Solarisation occurs with large x-ray exposures.

(d) Starts with a density of zero.

(e) The straight-line portion is the area best used for diagnostic purposes.

A3 (a) False – the characteristic curve is film density plotted against the $\log_{10}$ of exposure.

(b) False.

(c) True – solarisation occurs when a large exposure causes a reduction in density.

(d) True.

(e) True.

 Q4 Are the following statements regarding film density true or false?

(a) Film density is a measure of the blackness of a film.

(b) Film density is calculated as $\log_{10}$ (transmitted light intensity divided by incident light intensity).

(c) Film density is calculated as $\log_{10}$ (incident light intensity divided by transmitted light intensity).

(d) The unit of film density is the candela.

(e) Film density has a useful range of 0.25–2.

A4 (a) True.

(b) False – it is calculated as $\log_{10}$ (incident light intensity divided by transmitted light intensity).

(c)   True.
(d)   False – film density is unitless.
(e)   True.

 Q5   Are the following statements regarding film density true or false?
(a)   If 10% of light is transmitted then the film density will be 1.
(b)   The density of double emulsion films is multiplicative.
(c)   It is inversely related to the number of photons reaching the film.
(d)   It is measured with a penetrameter.
(e)   It is inversely related to transmittance.

A5   (a)   True.
(b)   False.
(c)   False.
(d)   False.
(e)   True.

Film density is measured with a densitometer. A penetrameter is used to measure the kV of an x-ray beam. Transmittance is calculated as the light intensity transmitted through the film divided by the light intensity hitting the film.

 Q6   Are the following statements regarding film speed true or false?
(a)   Film speed is calculated as the reciprocal of the air kerma.
(b)   A fast film requires fewer x-rays to produce a given density.
(c)   Speed is dependent on the average grain size of the film.
(d)   Speed is dependent on the energy of x-rays.
(e)   A slow film requires fewer x-rays to produce a given density.

(A6)

(a) True.
(b) True.
(c) True.
(d) True.
(e) False.

Film speed is calculated as the reciprocal of the air kerma required to give a film density of 1. Air kerma is the amount of kinetic energy transferred to charged particles by the uncharged per unit mass of irradiated air. Kerma is an acronym – kinetic energy released per unit mass. A fast film requires fewer x-rays to produce a given density and a slow film requires more x-rays. Speed is dependent on the average grain size of the film and energy of x-rays, presence of an intensification screen, presence of a double-sided screen and phosphor material.

(Q7)

Are the following statements regarding the film gamma true or false?
(a) Film gamma is the slope of the linear portion of the characteristic curve of the film.
(b) It is governed by the average grain size of the film.
(c) It is directly proportional to the range of film grain sizes.
(d) A high film gamma produces a film with better contrast.
(e) The steeper the linear portion of the characteristic curve, the greater the film contrast.

(A7)

(a) True.
(b) False.
(c) True.
(d) True.
(e) True.

The film gamma is calculated from the slope of the linear portion of the characteristic curve of the film. Film gamma is due to the range of grain sizes of the film. The average grain size is related to the film speed. A higher film gamma produces a film with better contrast.

Q8 Are the following statements regarding film speed true or false?
(a) It can be used to compare the properties of two films.
(b) The relative speed of two films is calculated as the exposure required to produce a density of 1 on film A divided by the exposure required to produce a density of 1 on film B.
(c) It is unitless.
(d) It cannot be derived from the characteristic curve.
(e) It is not an important consideration when choosing the most appropriate film for a particular purpose.

A8 (a) True.
(b) True.
(c) True.
(d) False.
(e) False.

The film speed is the reciprocal of the air kerma required to give a film density of 1. High-speed screens require fewer x-rays to produce a density of 1 and therefore a lower patient dose is needed.

Q9 Are the following statements regarding the exposure latitude true or false?
(a) It has a typical range of 40 to 1.
(b) The film used in mammography has a wide latitude.
(c) The chest x-ray film has a wide latitude.
(d) It represents the air kerma required to produce densities within the range of 0.25 to 2.0.
(e) It represents a range of exposure factors.

A9 (a) True.
(b) False – mammography requires a low latitude and high contrast film.
(c) True.
(d) True.
(e) True.

(Q10) Are the following statements true or false? Film speed, gamma and fog are affected by:
(a) development time.
(b) developer concentration.
(c) optimised conditions for each type of film to maximise gamma and minimise fog.
(d) developer temperature.
(e) presence of an intensification screen.

(A10) (a) True.
(b) True.
(c) True.
(d) True.
(e) True.

(Q11) Are the following statements regarding film-screen combinations true or false?
(a) The spatial resolution of a film is not affected by grain size.
(b) Using intensifying screens decreases spatial resolution.
(c) Using a single sided film emulsion decreases spatial resolution.
(d) Using a thinner screen increases spatial resolution.
(e) Using a smaller phosphor particle size decreases spatial resolution.

(A11) (a) False.
(b) True.
(c) False.
(d) True.
(e) True.

The spatial resolution of a film is dependent on grain size and single screen films have a greater spatial resolution than double screen films.

Q12 Are the following statements regarding quantum mottle true or false?
(a) To see an image clearly the signal-to-noise ratio must be at least 3.
(b) The signal-to-noise ratio equals the number of x-ray photons absorbed divided by the standard deviation of the noise.
(c) Increasing the number of x-ray photons absorbed makes the image smoother.
(d) The distribution of photons hitting a detector is described by a Gaussian distribution.
(e) Quantum mottle is affected by factors other than the number of photons hitting a detector.

A12 (a) True.
(b) True.
(c) True.
(d) False – it is described by a Poisson distribution.
(e) False.

Q13 Are the following statements true or false? Quantum mottle is affected by the:
(a) number of absorbed x-ray photons.
(b) screen conversion efficiency.
(c) screen thickness.
(d) average energy of the photons absorbed by the emulsion.
(e) grain size of the film-screen.

A13 (a) True.
(b) True.
(c) True.
(d) False.
(e) False.

Quantum mottle is primarily affected by the number of x-rays hitting the film. Therefore the factors increasing the number of photons hitting the film will decrease quantum mottle.

Are the following statements true or false? Decreasing the kV when using film-screens with a constant film density will have the following effects:
(a)   increased mA.
(b)   decreased entrance surface dose.
(c)   increased film processing time.
(d)   decreased exposure time.
(e)   increased scatter.

 (a)   False.
(b)   False.
(c)   False.
(d)   False.
(e)   False – decreasing the kV in this circumstance would result in a decreased scatter.

 Are the following statements true or false? Film contrast is independent of the:
(a)   type of film-screen combination.
(b)   processing of the film.
(c)   film density.
(d)   film latitude.
(e)   film speed.

 (a)   False.
(b)   False.
(c)   False.
(d)   False.
(e)   False.

Film contrast is the observed density differences on a radiograph and is determined by the slope of the characteristic curve. Film contrast is inversely related to fog level and film latitude.

Q16 Are the following statements regarding patient dosimetry true or false?
(a) A dose area product meter is most commonly used.
(b) It is a legal requirement to record patient radiation dose.
(c) Shields are used where possible.
(d) The entrance surface dose is higher for an antero-posterior (AP) pelvis radiograph than for a lateral lumbar spine radiograph.
(e) Typical fluoroscopy dose rates are 1 μGy/second at the input phosphor.

A16 (a) True.
(b) True.
(c) True.
(d) False.
(e) True.

The lateral lumbar spine has an entrance surface dose of approximately three times higher than for an AP pelvis.

Q17 Are the following statements true or false? Techniques used to reduce patient dose include:
(a) using tube filtration.
(b) using a high kV.
(c) decreasing the object-to-film distance.
(d) compressing the tissue to be imaged.
(e) using rare earth screens.

A17 (a) True.
(b) True.
(c) True.
(d) True.
(e) True.

All the above are techniques to reduce patient dose.

Film development and processing

 Q1 Are the following statements regarding film processing true or false?
(a) Film development requires the conversion of silver metal to ions in the sensitivity specks.
(b) An oxidising agent is used.
(c) The film needs to be fixed before development.
(d) Poor fixation results in a brown film appearance.
(e) An acidic pH is used in fixation.

A1 (a) False.
(b) False.
(c) False.
(d) False.
(e) False.

Film is processed by development, fixing and washing, and finally drying. Film is developed in an alkaline solution with a developing agent, which reduces the silver ions to metallic silver. Poor washing leads to a brown layer of silver sulphide. The fixation solution is alkaline.

Q2 Are the following statements true or false? Increasing the temperature of the developing process:
(a) increases the film speed.
(b) increases the film gamma.
(c) can decrease the film gamma.
(d) has no effect on the characteristic curve of the film.
(e) decreases the film fog.

A2
(a) True.
(b) True.
(c) True.
(d) False.
(e) False.

Increasing the developer temperature increases the speed of the film processing chemical reactions, which has predictable effects on the characteristic curve of the film-screen combination. The film speed, fog level and film gamma are increased with increasing developer temperature. Increasing the developer temperature initially increases the film gamma. However, increasing the temperature further will result in a decreased film gamma.

Q3
Are the following statements regarding film processing true or false?
(a) It principally converts the latent image into a permanent visible image.
(b) The developer is an electron donor.
(c) The developer reduces silver ions to silver atoms.
(d) The developer usually has no effect on the majority of unexposed silver ions.
(e) Film fog is due to the developer reducing unexposed silver ions.

A3
(a) True.
(b) True – the developer is an electron donor in an alkaline solution.
(c) True – the developer reduces exposed silver ions to silver atoms at the sensitivity specks.
(d) True.
(e) True.

It usually has no effect on the majority of unexposed ions.

Q4 Are the following statements regarding silver recovery true or false?

(a) The electrolytic method is cheaper than metallic replacement.

(b) Fixer can be re-used in the electrolytic method.

(c) Silver is deposited onto the anode in the electrolytic method.

(d) Wash solution can be re-used with the metallic replacement method.

(e) Silver is produced as a precipitate in the metallic replacement method.

A4 (a) False – the metallic replacement method is cheaper and uses steel wool.

(b) True – it can be re-used but it is an expensive process.

(c) False – silver is deposited onto the cathode (95% pure).

(d) True.

(e) True – it is precipitated and removed as sludge. The fixer cannot be reused in the metallic replacement method.

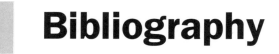

Bibliography

- Farr RF and Allisy-Roberts PJ (1997) *Physics for Medical Imaging*. WB Saunders Co., Philadelphia, PA.
- Curry TS, Dowdey JE and Murray RC (1990) *Christensen's Physics of Diagnostic Radiology* (4e). Lea & Febiger, Philadelphia, PA and London.
- Department of Health (1999) *Ionising Radiation Regulations 1999 [IRR 1999]*. DoH, London.
- Department of Health (2000) *Ionising Radiations (Medical Exposure) Regulations 2000 [IRMER 2000]*. DoH, London.

Index

Page numbers in *italics* refer to tables or illustrations.

133